CONQUERING MYSTERY PAIN

How Myofascial Release Can Help Heal YOU!

DR. JESSICA L. PAPA

CONTENTS

In the memory of my Grandmother Terry: Gram, I will be forever grateful that I spent the majority of my life with you. You are the backbone of who I am and the soul of what I have accomplished with Arancia PT. There is not a day that goes by when I do not think of you, miss you, or share your wisdom. I have been blessed to have you as my grandmother, role model, and cheerleader.

ACKNOWLEDGMENTS

*W*riting a book is harder than I thought and more rewarding than I could have ever imagined. Turning these thoughts and ideas into reality would never have been possible without the support of my parents, Carol and Robert Papa.

Mom and Dad, I know you can't pick your parents, but I am lucky to have ended up with you. Although our family life wasn't perfect (really, is anybody's?), you have taught me all of the important stuff: discipline, tough love, manners, respect, determination, and so much more. All of this has helped me succeed in life. I truly have no idea where I would be if I hadn't had your unshaking guidance, support, and shoulders to stand on.

The world is a better place thanks to people who want to develop and lead others. What makes it even better are the people who share the gift of their time to mentor future leaders. Thank you to everyone who strives to constantly grow and help others do the same.

To all the individuals I have had the opportunity to be led by: I want to say thank you for being the inspiration and foundation for this book. Special thanks to the colleagues and patients who have contributed and shared their stories within its pages. Storytelling has enormous power and it is my hope that these provided will help you to not feel alone-whatever you may be struggling with.

A very special thanks to my mentor, John F. Barnes, for introducing me to the world of Myofascial Release. John, I would like to express my gratitude from the bottom of my heart for your vital support and inspiration, without which this project would not have come to fruition. You have given me a tremendous amount of confidence in my work, as well as in my life.

A FOREWORD BY
JOHN F. BARNES, PT

*W*hat you're about to read is very important. The information in Dr. Jessica Papa's book, *Conquering Mystery Pain: How Myofascial Release Can Help Heal YOU!*, is especially important for those of you who have been suffering with pain, headaches, restriction of motion, fibromyalgia, athletic performance injuries, etc. I could go on, and on, and on with the labels. It turns out that traditional therapy and medicine have focused on symptoms and they give these symptoms labels. The problem is that symptomatic treatment is incomplete, and for most people will only give temporary relief because it doesn't resolve the cause. What I've found from my experience as a Physical Therapist for over 50 years is that it is the fascial system that is the cause for the vast majority of the problems that humans and animals suffer from.

I have been teaching my Myofascial Release seminars for over 45 years and have had the opportunity of training over 100,000 physicians and therapists from all over the world. Myofascial Release is now being used on millions of patients per month for decades now. There has not been one injury because the Myofascial Therapist does not use force!

I graduated from the University of Pennsylvania back in 1960 and I don't ever remember them mentioning the word "fascia." During anatomy class we dissected the cadavers and I remember the professor yelling at us to "clean that stuff off and throw it away!", referring to the fascia. Pretty much all healthcare professionals were taught that fascia was just unimportant packing material that covered muscles. I have been attacked for over 50 years because I dared to do something different. Basically, what I was told was that I had no research and I countered by saying, "You're right. I have no research, but I have results. You have research, but no results." Now, there is a voluminous amount of research that is backing up the importance of treating the fascial system.

The fascial system received nationwide attention in the past year. It was stated that science had made a mistake by studying dead people and by compressing the tissue together. With the advent of new laser optical technology, they can now see what I became aware of by treating patients for over 50 years ago, which is the 3-dimensional quality of the fascial system and its fluid component, the ground substance, which completely changes everyone's perspective.

The seminars that I teach are very large, and one day back in 2015 a beautiful, young therapist approached me with a brilliant smile to introduce herself. Jessica is an incredible Myofascial Release therapist, both for her intelligence and her ability to grasp the principles of Myofascial Release. She also has the skilled, sensitive touch of a therapeutic artist.

It turns out that all forms of therapy and exercise happen too quickly. Think about the frustration of not having anything more than temporary results. All the wonderful forms of massage are only rubbing over or digging into the tissue with force. Even light massage feels great, but it only produces short term effects. Mobilization, manipulation, muscle energy, modalities, and exercise are all in and out of the system too quickly, which means they are only affecting 20% of the fascial system.

The fascial system not only covers but interpenetrates every structure and system of our bodies all the way down to the cellular level. It is only through the artistic hands of the therapists, feeling into the individual's body, can they find out where your particular restrictions lie. Myofascial Release is truly individualized care!

Most therapists were taught protocols, sort of a "one size fits all" formula. There are over 7 billion people in the world. There are over 7 billion different fascial strain patterns. The art of Myofascial Release is to be able to feel where your pattern is and then apply the appropriate pressure and wait a sufficient amount of time for the release to occur. When a therapist engages the barrier, it's never done with brute force, but with gentle and firm pressure when done properly. We then wait. It takes 90-120 seconds to engage what's called the collagenous barrier. This is what has been missed in healthcare. We then wait another 3-5 minutes per barrier. There's a multitude of barriers in most humans and animals. The release is a sense of softening, like butter melting or taffy stretching. The therapist doesn't slide on the surface, but takes the slack out until they engage at the next barrier.

It is somewhere around the five minute period that a number of phenomena occur that are essential for healing, reduction of pain, and physiological health to occur. "Piezoelectricity" is a Greek word which means "pressure electricity." It is a well-known fact that our cells have a crystalline nature. When you place pressure into a crystal it creates an electrical flow. The sustained pressure of my Approach to Myofascial Release coupled with the time element, five minutes or longer per restriction, creates a bioelectrical flow in our body, which leads into mechanotransduction. Sustained mechanical pressure can also create biochemical changes within our bodies. Importantly, Myofascial Release produces interleukin 8, our body's own natural anti- inflammatory agent. These two occurrences, piezoelectricity and mechanotransduction, dovetail together and then Phase Transition takes place. This is the phenomena of ice transforming into water. In our bodies (although not ice) a similar occurrence happens. The solidification of the ground substance becomes more fluid, allowing the tissue to rehydrate and to glide, taking crushing pressure off pain-sensitive structures. When one human touches another human their vibratory rates are quite different on the molecular level, however with sustained pressure at the fascial restriction, the vibratory rates will become identical, creating resonance. Resonance is the very essence of my Approach to Myofascial Release. This is what I call a "Release." Release occurs both in the cranial area and throughout the body. Resonance, unfortunately, does not occur in other forms of therapy due to the sheer fact that these other forms of therapy are too quick, hence providing only temporary results. The good news is that Myofascial Release, coupled with various forms of therapy, massage, bodywork, energy techniques and exercise, will greatly enhance your effectiveness.

Myofascial Release can be used in a broad variety of settings for a wide range of diagnoses, such as back pain, cervical pain, headaches, spasm/spasticity, chronic pain, carpal tunnel, fibromyalgia, scoliosis, sports injuries, Women's Health issues, disc problems, sciatica, and TMJ.

Listen carefully to Dr. Jess' perspective. It will give you the hope of possibly resolving the problems that you've been imprisoned by for too long of a time. Best of luck!

John F. Barnes, PT
Myofascial Release Treatment Centers
www.MyofascialRelease.com
800-327-2425

INTRODUCTION

*L*et's talk pain. Pain comes in many forms, yet can be a difficult topic to grasp. Pain serves one purpose: it tells your body that this is not okay and gives you the instinct to withdraw. But, what if you don't know why your body is feeling that pain? How do you run when you do not know where to run from?

What if, when you seek guidance and safety, you are only told to ignore it? For many people, this has become a part of their life. For me, this is not an option. There is always a reason for pain and I am here to help you get to the bottom of it. I cannot begin to tell you how many times I've had patients and prospective patients come to me with a pain that they have not yet been able to find relief for, despite years of trying. Ultimately, they are concerned about losing mobility and worry they will not be able to do the things they once used to.

These patients often have had diagnostic imaging (MRI/ X- ray/ CT-scan) ordered by their general practitioners, but when their doctor evaluates the results they are often told that there is nothing wrong with them. All of this, despite the fact that their pain is still present. Instead of further investigation, they are often told to "rest" and come back in a few weeks.

The issue here is twofold: first, the patient's pain or discomfort is being completely ignored and overlooked; second, the doctor is not taking into account the very real possibility that the source of the patient's pain lies in the fascial system. The fascial system, which makes up 70% of the human body, cannot be seen; it doesn't show up on any diagnostic image.

For this reason, any issue originating within this system may be completely written off. Mystery pain is just an injury that has not yet been identified. Ignoring an entire system of tissue that runs through the whole body can, and does, result in people living with pain indefinitely and unnecessarily. This affects their everyday life, and ultimately, their quality of life.

In order to fully disclose the intimate relationship I have with mystery pain and explain why I can help you in discovering yours, I need to bring you back to one of the most agonizing periods of my life. This was a phase of my journey when pain was all that I knew and all that I could see, but had no way of identifying the actual reason I was suffering.

Much like my patients who deal with chronic mystery pain, my life has been divided into two: the time before the injury and the time after. My journey as a Physical Therapist began in 2013 when I was a brand new graduate. I entered the medical profession with fresh eyes and was full of enthusiasm. On top of my new career, I had a new husband. We had moved into a beautiful home, a two minute walk from the beach in Rhode Island. Our pups kept us company in our free hours, often visiting the ocean and finding new trails to hike. The world seemed to offer an endless supply of opportunity and I relished every second of it, running from one goal to the next.

A few years into my career I was hired as a Doctor of Physical Therapy in a small, mom-and-pop style clinic. It was not far from the hospital where I had first started my career and felt like a fantastic fit. It was there that I first discovered my love of physical therapy, especially when working one-on-one with patients, and met some of the physical therapists who I still find inspiration with to this day. At the hospital, I built long-lasting relationships and connections with patients and colleagues who have been integral pieces of my puzzle. Unfortunately, the enthusiasm that I had entered the position with quickly began to wane as I became disinterested with the monotony and uninventive tools I had at my disposal.

I can still remember the first time I felt the passion leave my work. I was sitting at my desk at the beginning of my day, steaming mug of coffee beside me and my computer booting up. My boss had instructed my fellow therapists and me to fill out a schedule before beginning appointments. We were expected to account for our time with each patient, planning the treatment we would be giving. All of this, before having met some of the patients even once. My boss had implemented a system in which we would give our rehabilitation technicians a plan for the patients, even if they hadn't been seen or examined, so that we, the therapists, would have more time for documentation. Emphasis was put on maximizing how many patients we could see, quickly moving through appointments with efficiency, not compassion.

I so badly wanted to call my Grandmother, my biggest supporter and friend, to discuss how much I hated what I was doing, yet I could not quite pinpoint exactly why I was feeling that way. I was supposed to be happy, wasn't I? Everything was going according to plan. This was the first sign that not all was healthy in my life.

Soon I was simply going through the motions; my days becoming longer and longer as my career began to lose the luster I once thought it had. I stopped seeing the differences I once believed I made in my patients' lives, and it took a toll on me. Mondays were dreaded. Tuesdays were to be conquered. Wednesdays made me sick. Thursdays dragged on. By the time I forced myself into work on Fridays, I barely felt like the young, enthusiastic professional I had begun the job as.

As unbearable as my work life had become, home was worse. Though I was increasingly unfulfilled at work, I was safe. I was competent. I was, at the very least, in control. My marriage had begun to fall apart before my very eyes, and the rest of my life followed suit. Just as the body cannot take trauma after trauma without showing signs of injury, you cannot hide the bruises of a broken heart.

We met and fell in love shortly after high school when we were both eighteen. After two years of dating, he left to serve in the military. When he came back, he was not the man I had said goodbye to. Despite my parents' misgivings, we were married three years later, eager to continue on to the next chapter in our lives.

In hindsight, there were many signs that I was blinded to. We were young, had spent a majority of our relationship long distance, and really did not know each other at the depth that we should have before making the commitment of marriage. I ignored all of this, even though my family did not. At the time, there was no way for me to diagnose the source of all the pain that had piled up within me. It only got worse.

This, and more, led me to sign up for a continuing education class on a whim, desperate for change. It was a class that explored Myofascial Release by John F. Barnes. I can still remember the feeling of the glossy mailer in my hands as I read through the list of classes that would be offered, breathing in the distinct smell of brochure ink. Each class looked more exciting than the last. I lingered on that mailer longer than I had paused to breathe in the morning air that day.

Hope bubbled within me; a feeling that had been all too absent in recent months. Passion had once again found a place in my life after that class. Passion, not a frantic search for distraction, but genuine, slow-burning fervor. I knew, even then, that what I had been missing was near.

In Phoenix, Arizona I discovered not only my professional passion, but also the cure for the unidentified illness within my personal life. Myofascial Release became the therapy upon which I would build my practice. It would become the tool that would heal the many patients that would pass through my office, and the passion that I would eventually wish to share. I learned, through Myofascial Release, why I was hurting and how to begin healing.

At one time I regretted making the decisions that lead me to that place where so much pain came into my life, but now I have a different mindset. Every choice you make and every step you take in life, even if it is a stumble, has a purpose. Every moment of growing pain I went through over the course of my ill-fated marriage brought me closer to my passion, to this amazing, fulfilling career. My unwillingness to settle gave me the drive to change and my injuries gave me the perspective I needed in order to recognize when others are hurt.

No, you are not alone. Everyone has a secret pain, whether it may be physical or emotional, including me. With Myofascial Release, not only can we find the solution to your physical pain, but get to the source of the emotional stagnation that you may be suffering, as well. Together we can uncover, heal, and conquer.

WHAT IS MYOFASCIAL RELEASE?

*"Failure to recognize the importance of fascia with respect
to the body's structure and movement helps explain many
of the poor or temporary results achieved with standard
treatment." - John F. Barnes, PT*

*M*yofascial Release is an innovative physical therapy that has been practiced in its modern form since the 1960s. It is a therapy that involves the gentle application of pressure at various points of restriction in the fascia in order to relieve pain or restore motion. Not well understood, it has only found popularity within the last decade. Due to this popularity, we have finally seen a huge amount of sorely needed research being conducted.

John F. Barnes, a Physical Therapist and licensed Massage Therapist, is one of the most influential persons in the therapeutic profession in this century. He has been instrumental in the development and popularization of the Myofascial Release Approach as a therapy for mystery pain and other ailments. Because of this, he is often referred to as the Father of Myofascial Release.

He is recognizable not only in medical circles, but also to laypeople thanks to 2018's national breaking news about the fascial system, which brought to light the fact that research up to that point had been inaccurate at best. The inaccuracies were found to be caused by the fact that all observations of fascia had been done on dead tissue, rather than on living patients.

Using laser technology, researchers are now able to see clearer images of fascia and have taken great strides to further our understanding of its function. In addition, this research has confirmed the validity of the work Barnes has been doing over the last 50 years, namely treating the fascial system as a three-dimensional quality web, alive with fluid.

He is still active in educating the current generation of therapists, myself included, through his company, Myofascial Release Seminars. I have been one of over 100,000 therapists and physicians who have been educated at the cutting edge of this therapy; learning the ins and outs of helping people of all ages and backgrounds in finding the root of their pain, as well as treating them mind, body, and soul.

FIRST THING'S FIRST: FASCIA

"Sometimes you don't realize the weight of something you've been carrying until you feel the weight of its release." - Anonymous

The very basis of Myofascial Release (MFR) is identifying and treating restrictions within the little-known tissue called fascia. If you have never heard of fascia, you are not alone. Very few people are aware that there is a tissue that covers more of you than your skin, and that it can be the source of many problems and issues you may be facing in your daily life. Let's explore, together, what fascia is in context of your body and how it can be affecting you everywhere, from the strange tingling in your feet to the tension headaches in your skull.

Fascia is a thin layer of connective tissue that lays over your muscles and extends all the way down to the cellular level of the body. It covers each organ, nerve, muscle, bone, and vein. The entirety of fascia is called the fascial system and when fascia is restricted it is often referred to as "the straight jacket."

This epithet is derived from the fact that there is not a square inch of your body that does not have an overlay of fascial tissue. So, when your fascia cannot move freely, it is effectively binding you to your body. It becomes a trap that you cannot escape. In short, from the tip-top of your head to the bottom of your toes, fascia covers your entire being.

This interesting part of your anatomy is composed of two types of fibers: collagenous fibers, which are very tough and have little stretchability; and elastic fibers, which are stretchable. It lies over your muscles and goes all the way down to the cellular level without interruption. It is considered to be a major system and organ known as the "interstitia."

The interstitia is the only system that surrounds and invades every other tissue and organ of the body, including nerves, vessels, muscles, and bones. Interestingly, fascia is more dense in some areas than others, depending on where in the body it is located.

My favorite analogy when explaining fascia is that of an orange. When we peel an orange, it easily separates into slices that are divided by a sturdy, transparent tissue. The tissue in the orange sections is similar to the fascia under our skin. The slices of oranges are held together under the thick, outer skin by a thin, white layer of pith, which is analogous to the superficial fascial layers that run throughout our bodies. In the very center of the orange there is a long, white center that keeps the orange connected and intact until it's pulled off or the slices are physically separated. This center connector is much like the deeper fascial layer beneath our skin. These deeper fascial layers hold our muscles and organs apart from one another, yet simultaneously hold them together in the same layer underneath the skin.

This extensive tissue serves multiple important functions as well, including the stabilization and connection of your various muscles and other tissues. If you were to peek beneath your skin, you would see it working constantly to keep you moving and functioning properly.

Because of the overreaching nature of your fascial system, when damage occurs there is a long string of consequences throughout your many other systems. It is vulnerable for the exact reason it is so very strong: it is everywhere.

Functionally, fascia allows the body to resist mechanical stresses, both internally and externally. It also provides a sliding and gliding environment for muscles, suspends organs in their proper place, transmits movement from muscles to the bones they are attached to, and provides a supportive and movable wrapping for nerves and blood vessels as they pass through and between muscles. Of course, if fascia is not acting and reacting properly, you can begin to experience disorders of any one of these functions.

When healthy, fascia is structured in a way that looks relaxed and wavy in configuration. It should be able to move and change with the rest of the body easily and without resistance. When an injury occurs and the physicality of fascia is altered through trauma, emotional or physical, it loses the pliable characteristics that are so very important to its function.

The fascia can "bunch up" when patterns are broken and over adjusting occurs at the point of damage. When this happens, the layers of fascia are no longer uniform and can instead form knots, similar to those in a piece of lumber. These knots eventually restrict motion and can render certain movements impossible.

This is when you see and feel fascia change in a noticeable way. It can feel hot, hard or tender, and rigid. Dehydrated, the tissues no longer glide along each other easily; it becomes more like beef jerky, immobile and tough. Fascial malfunction will begin to become more and more evident as the fascia is pulled tight or stretched beyond its abilities in places where it was not meant to stretch at all. This results in tissue restriction, decreased mobility, and ultimately, pain.

The main instigator of these irregularities is trauma. For our purposes, the term "trauma" describes events such as surgery, accidents, injury, repetitive activities, stress, and postural patterns. At the point of injury or trauma, fibers of the fascia become restricted and in turn, prevent fluid from passing through the fascial system the way that it should, as described above. This produces an incredible amount of tensile pressure.

We talk a lot about how fascia is integral in all parts of our body. Our brain is no exception. Dura, or the specific fascia that encompasses the brain and adjoining central nervous system, has an important job. When healthy, the dura keeps the flow of oxygen to our cells and neurotransmitters unimpeded, and detoxes within those areas. As expected, when those functions are disrupted by pressure or injury, you are left with physiological illness, depression, anxiety, and nerve pain. Due to the overarching importance of the dura, some speculate that this also triggers our fight-or-flight response, which we will explore in detail later.

Keeping all of this in mind, let's explore the physicality behind this phenomenon. For example, Gerald H. Pollack, PhD at the University of Washington, provided a comprehensive study that probed into the specialized method that fluid moves through the fascial system, and why the restriction of fluid through the system is so damaging in his book, *The Fourth Phase of Water: Beyond Solid, Liquid and Vapor* (2014).

Dr. Pollock discovered that, despite the common conception that water exists in three states of matter (liquid, ice, and vapor), there is actually a fourth option: liquid crystal. Liquid crystal has characteristics of both a solid and a liquid, and has the capability to change. Fascia's properties are very similar to that of liquid crystal, making them almost synonymous, and thus there is a direct scientific connection (Pollack, 2014).

Pressure and restriction of fluid will cause pain. This pain, while often immense, is not something that will be evident in X-rays or MRI tests. As a result, many patients who experience pain that cannot be explained by an obvious injury through imaging are often overlooked by medical practitioners who do not have training in MFR. The pain then remains unchecked and untreated. Misdiagnosis runs rampant within the medical community pertaining to the particular subject of myofascial pain.

To further exacerbate this issue within pain management, the point of discomfort that a patient may be experiencing is often far from the true location of the fascial damage. Fluid restriction and points of stress can, and very often, affect the entire body. We likened fascia to a web for a reason. For example, patients may identify pain in their right shoulder when they are actually experiencing fascial abnormality at a surgery site on their back which had been operated on many years before.

The most simple way to illustrate the reasoning behind all of this is in the way Dr. Pollock himself describes fascia. According to him, we are not simply covered by fascia, we are in fact, "fascial beings." It is a matrix, and by its very nature, adapts to us at the same time that we change because of it. There is no end to the immersive influence it has over us and all functions that make our lives possible.

For many, many years physical therapists, like John F. Barnes, who knew this to be true were invalidated by faulty and insufficient research. The issue was that we did not have accurate modeling of the human body when healthy and alive. Dr. Jean- Claude Guimberteau, a French hand and plastic surgeon, remedied this when in 2005 he updated the model of human anatomy through his groundbreaking research (*Strolling Under the Skin*, 2006).

With visual evidence, he was able to show exactly what fascial tissue actually looks like on a living human. This has become the irrefutable corroboration that John F. Barnes and Dr. Pollock needed to show that fascia is a completely integrated part of the body.

Damage to fascia is much harder to remedy than a topical injury because of the static state of the tissue, even if it is identified and diagnosed. No amount of stretching, heating, icing, or exercise will lessen pain that stems from fascial damage because those conventional methods of pain alleviation do not address the source of the injury. Because of this, it can be the cause of chronic pain.

Your chronic pain is present for a reason. Thanks to the researchers and physical therapists who have dedicated their lives to the study of fascia, you have a chance of not only identifying the reason for it, but also a treatment. Myofascial Release has been built on this fact, now it is up to the patient to utilize it.

THE PRACTICE OF
MYOFASCIAL RELEASE

*N*ow that we have a baseline understanding of what fascia is and how it pertains to your body, let's explore the actual science behind Myofascial Release and how it is practiced within the medical community.

In medical school, you are taught to look at the human body as broken and in need of repair. All of our parts are divided into convenient systems, such as the Cardiovascular System, the Lymphatic System, the Musculoskeletal System, and more, losing much of the connectivity that is so innate in our makeup. Similar to how a mechanic looks at a car, doctors are taught to locate the source of an issue, diagnose it, look for the steps to repair it, and do so. The problem here is that physicians and therapists are being taught to use a linear line of logic on a nonlinear system.

The protocols, routines, and formulas that work for most individuals are being taught, in some spaces, to be considered a solution for all. In physical therapy, this is not the case. We are taught to look at the body as if we have never seen one before. For every diagnosis and symptomatic complex, there are billions of possible fascial restrictions that can cause what we think of as symptoms.

No wonder people with unexplained pain are often only given temporary relief from their pain. Just because you can't see it, does not mean that it is not there! When we hold ourselves and others to a higher standard of care, of looking at each body and pain as a new mystery to uncover and treat, we are able to do better for each patient that we come in contact with.

Sometimes this requires us to "soften our focus," which is why I perform a thorough postural assessment when I receive a new patient. I take photos from four different perspectives at the beginning of the patient's session. Then, I share the photos with them, and show them where they are spilling forward, backward, or in any other direction. Once I have explained to the patient where their posture is deviating, I always begin treatment by addressing pelvic alignment. I do this while the patient is standing so that I can see the way they hold their bodies while gravity is in place, weighing them down.

This standard of care allows me to begin treatment by taking into account a very basic part of a patient's life. I can identify immediately where there is a need for correction and begin to address it. No two people carry themselves in the same exact way, resulting in a unique correction for each patient right off the bat. The customization does not stop there.

Something to keep in mind when you are attempting to locate the source of discomfort is that we all perform different repetitive activities throughout the course of a day, week, month, and year. I am talking about the way you sit in your favorite work chair or how you perform the same activities at the gym. Over time, our bodies start to compensate and stiffness, loss of motion, and pain can creep in. This should be the first stop when we are looking for clues.

This is an example of how I, as a Myofascial Release Expert, am trained to treat the symptoms, but look elsewhere for the root cause. Instead of treating just the symptomatic area, pieces and parts, I treat the whole person, mind and body. Neck pain may be stemming from a birthing injury or trauma. A fall you had well over ten years ago can now cause jaw pain and headaches. Back strain can be the root cause of your knee discomfort.

You can see a clear difference between MFR and traditional therapy in practice, as well. Authentic John F. Barnes Myofascial Release has three pillars: Unwinding, Rebounding, and structural work. All three are used in varying amounts and ways to produce unique results for unique patients.

During Unwinding, the goal is for the patient to coerce the mind to let go of its grasp on the trauma and stressors. When this is achieved, the body is able to authentically move, or unwind. This then kickstarts the healing process and the release of fascial restrictions, altering the habitual muscular "holding patterns" that the body has adapted. It is important to note that your therapist cannot unwind you; only the patient can truly achieve this. By doing so, you can reproduce space where trauma has occurred.

When you achieve Unwinding, forces such as gravity no longer have bearing on your fascia and other symptoms. The therapist aiding you can then help you move past trauma in a physical sense, allowing your responses to move past the freeze cycle.

Another hallmark of MFR that will become a fixture during your treatment is a rhythmic oscillatory motion called Rebounding. Its main purpose is that of an assessment tool. It helps the therapist recognize where there is a need for structural work. It is also used on people who have a difficult time letting go of their holding patterns, which is common in new patients. The therapist will usually lay the patient down on the table, and while not using force, will perform the motion, creating minimal dialogue between you, taking your lead and following your body's motion. Rebounding is incredibly important due to the twofold purpose that it serves the patient, both as a relaxation tool and as an assessment tool to begin their treatment.

Myofascial Release can relieve that pressure in your body and allow it to return to equilibrium. Often, when people have myofascial occipital condyle releases, or cranial work, their depression lifts, anxiety lessens, and the person is able to return to a more healthy state of peace and tranquility (Barnes, n.d.).

Now, those who are in need of physical therapy may very well need other treatment, as well. Chiropractic adjustments can work in tandem with MFR to create longer-lasting effects. In order to demonstrate why,

I would like for you to picture an old fashioned tent, the type with a central pole and one large piece of canvas. It should look like a large triangle when set up. Imagine that the pole is your skeletal system, and the ropes holding the canvas down with tension, is your fascia. Just as the ropes help keep the tent upright and stable, so does your fascia. If you suffer from fascial restrictions, or your ropes are tangled and have slack, your bones can become unaligned.

Let's say that you have a holding pattern in your shoulder from an injury and it is causing you discomfort in your neck. If you visit a chiropractor, they will attempt to adjust the spine. This may work temporarily, but if the holding pattern in your shoulders is not adjusted, the benefits will not last, just as the tent will fall if the ropes are not adjusted to the height or position of the central pole. Tissue moves bone, and it has the potential to put up to 2,000 pounds per square inch of pressure on pain-sensitive structures.

When fascia is injured, there is a common misconception that one must treat it as a muscle injury, and often people are advised to ice the site. This can be just as ineffectual as treating the spine without the fascia. When connective tissue gets cold, it loses its elasticity and the interstitial fluid that fills all the spaces between the body structures thickens, and in so, you are achieving the worst state for your fascia possible when injured.

Dr. Gabe Mirkin, the doctor who coined the RICE (Rest, Ice, Compression, Elevation) method, states when you apply ice to reduce swelling, it constricts blood vessels near the injury and thus shuts off the flow of blood that carries the macrophages that release IGF-1 to repair the injured tissue. Your blood vessels won't reopen for many hours after the application of ice. This decrease in blood supply can cause the tissue to die, leading to permanent damage.

Dr. Mirken, in lieu of this, recommends that if pain is acute, apply ice only as a temporary, short term measure. He adds that, if more than six hours have passed after an injury, there is no reason to apply ice, rather compression over the injury is beneficial.

Timing also plays an important role in the practice of MFR. As we talked about, new research has shown that fascia reaches all the way down to the cellular level. This makes it crucial for the therapist to hold each and every technique for a minimum of five minutes. It is only at the five minute mark that interleukin 8 and 1B are released in the body.

Interleukin 8 is our body's natural anti-inflammatory fighter. Research has demonstrated the significant role that inflammation plays in physical reparation. At the point that inflammation and other irritant has been resolved, ground substance within fascia becomes solid, when it is meant to be in a fluid state. When solidification takes place, your body can no longer heal and this eventually leads to restrictions. These restrictions become the mystery or misdiagnosed pain that is so often present in patients (Meltzer et al., 2010).

As our bodies become better understood, inflammation has been shown more and more to be the root of most, if not all, diseases, which is why the triggering of these chemicals is so important in pain resolution. Alzheimer's, heart disease, and more can be traced back to chronic inflammation, and the more that we conduct studies, the more sure the medical community becomes of this fact. When your body experiences MFR and releases this chemical, it not only helps with the pain that is caused by the actual inflammation, but also the root cause of the inflammation itself.

When a MFR therapist begins a session, the first hold will start a sequence of events that will eventually lead to a resolution that our bodies crave. First, the patient's body begins to produce piezoelectricity. "Piezoelectricity" is a Greek word that translates to "pressure electricity," which is fitting in this context.

The cells of our body have a crystalline nature, and when you put pressure into a crystal it generates an electrical flow. So, in our body, what occurs is a bio-electric flow. This is then coupled with a phenomenon called "mechanotransduction." Our mechanical pressure, around the five-minute mark, begins to produce a biochemical, hormonal effect at the cellular level (Nelson and Bissell, 2006).

Now, the process of mechanotransduction is imperative to the method of Myofascial Release, as well. This is when physical energy or force sets into motion the generation of biochemical responses. In earlier hypothesis, it was thought that this generation was only due to biochemistry and genetic action at the cellular level. New research shows that not only does mechanotransduction play a part, but the fascia outside of the cell affects the internal physicality of the cell when pressure is applied. This may be the origin of malignancies (Oschman, n.d.).

Next, we move into phase transition, which is the phenomenon where ice transforms into water. During this phase, piezoelectricity and mechanotransduction work together. The solidified or dehydrated ground substance of fascia, with sustained pressure, becomes more fluid, allowing the tissue to rehydrate and to glide, taking crushing pressure off pain-sensitive structures.

Obviously, in our body, it's not ice; instead it is the solidification of the fluid component of the fascial system. This is referred to as "ground substance," which creates that before-mentioned crushing pressure on pain-sensitive structures. It triggers a chaotic period during the phase transition. It is during this chaotic period where change, growth, and healing can occur.

The chaos period is an interesting concept that MFR embraces, when other forms of medicine refuse to. Everything in traditional medicine and therapy insists upon order. Chaos Theory speculates that healing cannot occur in a controlled and orderly way. It states that nature goes through a continuous cycle of periods that alternate between order and chaos. The chaos period that is achieved during MFR is when reorganization of this cycle takes place, allowing for ice to transform into water, or in our terms, solidified ground substance of the fascial system is able to transform into a more gelatinous, fluid state.

Ultimately, at the end of the hold resonance is achieved. Researchers report, in several studies on vibration and biomagnetic energy that the human body emits, that when one human touches another, vibratory rates can differ at the molecular level. Researchers, however, have also found that with sustained pressure on the fascial restriction site, the vibratory rates of two bodies will become identical, creating resonance.

Resonance is the essence of the JFB-MFR approach. Researchers show that when resonance is reached it occurs locally, as well as vibrating distantly throughout the living crystal matriculants of fascia in the cranial area, as well as all the other far reaches of the human body (Bordoni and Zanier, 2014). Resonance, unfortunately, is not achieved with other forms of therapy because the movements and pressure are performed far too quickly, thus achieving only temporary results. These phenomena allow the tissue, which has solidified and produced crushing pressure, to start to rehydrate and become capable of gliding again. This takes the pressure off of pain-sensitive structures to enable proper function and elimination of pain.

MYOFASCIAL RELEASE
IN ACTION

*S*o, what is Myofascial Release like in action? In the most simple of terms, light pressure is placed on the points of tension, working the damaged tissue gently. It can be used on very small, localized areas, as well as larger areas, such as the torso, arms, and legs. This technique provides a new and fundamental way of accessing the consciousness of the body and mind.

When a person becomes an engaged participant in their therapy, a transformation of mind and body occurs, known as Enlightened Movement. Musculoskeletal and neurochemical influences create soft tissue restrictions in the mind and body. The body stores stress and soft tissue pain in certain patterns known as trigger points, muscle spasms, tension, headaches, etc. You have likely identified this in yourself, and your body's own method of storing accumulated pressure. Holding these patterns of tension for long periods causes the fascial system to adaptively shorten and puts immense pressure on the entire body, including your nerves, muscles, and vascular structure. In the long run, this lessens your tolerance to life stress and causes physical pain. Rather than looking at symptoms as entities in and of themselves, which must be manipulated, medicated, or "fixed," therapists trained in authentic Myofascial Release look for the cause and seek to establish balance within the body.

WHAT TO EXPECT
ON THE TABLE

"Let go of expectations and let go of attachment to outcomes." -*Deepak Chopra*

At this point, you may be wondering why John F. Barnes Myofascial Release works, where other therapies do not. The fascial system is made up of microtubules and marries all the other structures of the body, such as veins, nerves, other body systems (Lymphatic System, Endocrine System, etc.). It does not just exist in one place. It penetrates every cell, from the brain to the skin. Restrictions or adhesions affect the fascial system by binding it down, causing thickening, hardening, and increased pressure. As we discussed, this is where pain comes in.

JFB-MFR has been developing and refining MFR over the past 40 years to make this approach the most advanced and effective hands-on care available, particularly for patients who have not responded to traditional medical or surgical interventions. Once the fascial system is addressed, these same patients can begin to make progress in a matter of weeks with intensive MFR treatments, and are on their way to a pain-free, active lifestyle.

If you suffer from unexplained pain or discomfort, MFR is likely right for you. Knowing this, let us consider what to expect when you visit a practitioner of this therapy. While no two sessions will look the same, you can expect your therapist to adhere to utilize a basic set of principles.

All patients are unique and will have an experience that is individual to them. Your therapist will treat you and your pain according to what makes you comfortable, as well as providing advice. Your therapist may test the waters a bit and nudge you out of your comfort zone, where true growth and change take place. By following any or all of the suggestions, you can optimize the healing potential within you, meaning that your response to each treatment will be maximized. Repetition deepens the releases and the more you dive into your own experience, the more you will realize these effects. Your therapist is there to support you on your journey. They should guide and facilitate you in a non-forceful, creative, and effective manner.

No two sessions will look alike between practices or therapists. This is, therefore, a whole-body approach to evaluation and treatment. The therapist needs to use skin-to-skin contact to provide the friction interface needed in order to release the fascia effectively. Release of these fascial restrictions includes specific, specialized, manual techniques of holding the tissue for a minimum of 90 to 120 seconds to allow biome-chanical reactions to begin. Full release of the restriction may take five minutes or longer. Successive releases, through each layer, also require this time element. This approach is successful because we treat a system in the body that no one else treats: the fascial system.

The Fascial Voice Experience Scan takes place over your body before, during, and after treatment. During this, your therapist will request that you alert them if you are feeling areas of heat, tingling, or tightness. They look for reddened areas and other abnormalities, also known as the Vasomotor Response, where tissue becomes red as blood comes to the surface. It is imperative that you report any findings at the next treatment session. This provides the therapist with important information about areas that may need treatment.

Breathwork is another important piece of your treatment. Breathe into your area of pain or the area being treated when cued by the therapist. Visualize a tube going straight to that area and breathe through the tube into the pain, or into the part of your body that is being stretched and compressed.

In addition to this, always be aware. You should sink your awareness into the pain through feeling, not thought. Allow the area to feel like sinking sand. Do this by lending your consciousness to the inside of your body. In that same area, scan your whole body to feel the connections to other areas. Ask yourself, "Where does this connect internally?" Allow those areas to soften like butter melting or taffy pulling. Imagine more space in that area. And of course, provide feedback at your next session.

Keeping this in mind, relaxation and comfort is a key component to MFR. In order for the therapist to work effectively, the patient must be in a state that allows that. If this is achieved, the patient's health, posture, flexibility, and circulation have a much better chance of improving. As a direct result, they will experience their pain and muscle tension being alleviated. It is the wisdom of your body, listen to it.

When you move through treatment, be aware that your progress may not be a straight line towards your goal. Instead, it can come in a zigzag. A flare-up can occur and set you back at any moment. Allow yourself to be frustrated, even mourn your lost time, but do not give up. Healing is a journey that takes you through many mountains and valleys. Walk with your therapist and rejoice at every turn point. No matter what, you are moving forward.

Have goals in mind. Then, make an effort to support yourself in accomplishing them. I remind my patients that these goals are adaptable, should be something you enjoy, and reward yourself often. Once you have done this, you can look at pain in a new light. Pain can become your friend; it can become your teacher. It can show you where something is wrong and point you in the direction of healing.

THE LAST NIGHT
OF MY OLD LIFE

"It is a fundamental law of human nature, that you only get stronger by doing difficult things."- Robert Greene

*I*t all started with the tapping. In the quiet moments, when you lie down with the person you love and have idle conversation, where you should feel safe, he would tap. If I said something he disagreed with, he would tap. If we were at a party and the conversation steered toward a discussion he disapproved of, he would tap. At home, making dinner, if I responded to a question in a way he did not like, he would tap. On the forehead, the shoulder, the chest, anywhere he could reach, he would tap.

With just enough force to move my body one way or the other, his taps would continue through the day, through the years, through our marriage. Like a rhythmic, incessant reminder that I was wrong. My only defense was to pretend that they did not bother me. In fact, I would pretend not to feel them at all.

That only made things worse. If I left the room, he would follow. If I was cornered, he would take my keys away so I couldn't leave at all. He would hold me there, always tapping, until I finally did or said what he wanted. Even then, he would tap.

There would be no more tapping. The decision had barely been made when my life changed in a single night. For better or worse, it was the last night of my old life. I had just fallen into the comfortable haze of sleep when I heard the squeaking of our front door. He came in to the room ready for a fight. Now, it seems silly to argue so heatedly over clothes being folded. In that moment though, it felt like the most important fight we could ever have.

The fight reached its climax in the usual way, with me cornered in the room. He guarded the door like a bloodhound, having taken my keys and my phone. What was different that night was that instead of the tapping, I was on the bed being smothered by a pillow.

I can still remember the way the weight of his body over mine pushed the air from me. The pillow was so tight over my face that I couldn't draw a deep breath, and slowly, I could feel the air in my lungs leach out of me, forcing the weight to grow heavier and heavier.

Panicked, I pushed against him with all my strength, using my legs wedged under him to force some space between us. I just needed air. He pushed the pillow down even tighter. Little by little, I became weaker. With no air to fuel me, I knew that my time was limited.

A little voice in my head fought past the frantic thoughts of impending doom. *How could he do this to me? What did I do wrong? Why does the love of my life, my husband, want to hurt me?* Just as I started to accept the possibility that he truly wished to suffocate me, he finally released me.

He kicked me off the edge of the bed so that I landed harshly on the floor. I was in shock. My body began to shake, tremors taking over my being. I felt as if I was no longer in the body I had been in before he reached out to me. Numb and heartbroken, I rocked back and forth, attempting to wrap my head around what had just happened, not only to me, but to my marriage.

You have suffered enough. You are okay now, but you have to leave. You are not safe here. It was as if my grandmother was there with her reassuring words, pulling me from the darkest of places. This was not the last time I was with my husband, but it was one of the last.

The thought of my Gram kept me grounded over the course of that terrible night. My parents had been lucky, and both of my grandmothers lived on the street directly behind our home when I was young and my mother struggled with her health. My grandmothers picked up what slack they could. I was especially close with my maternal grandmother, Grandma Terry. Gram was present in the way that I yearned for in my mother and provided an immense amount of comfort and support. I clung to her presence just as tightly as I clung to my legs as I sat there curled into a ball, rocking back and forth.

I didn't know it then, but one of the hardest things to do in my entire life was toward the end of hers. Years later I sat at the edge of her bed, holding her familiar hand in mine, choking back tears, when I asked for wisdom that I did not have. It was then that I finally revealed to her the awful secret I had been keeping.

She was my biggest fan. Telling her that I had failed, that my marriage was not working, and that I was ready to quit was my biggest fear, but she was a smart woman. She knew me better than I knew myself, she just needed me to say the words. Finally I did. I explained to her how my husband had changed, that life had gotten so hard, and even though I had a stubborn wish to stay married, I had left and never told her because I didn't want to disappoint her, ever. I poured my heart out to her in a way that I wish I had much, much sooner.

She was 95, but as smart as a tack. She held me in her arms the way she had held me as a child, and began to rock me. This rocking comforted me the way I could not comfort myself when I was alone, the sting of my ex-husband's touch still fresh on my neck. I could see the sadness in her eyes and her heart, but that embrace showed me that her sadness was not for my decisions, it was for the pain I was in.

She rocked me and told me, "You are my strong girl, you will be fine. I love you, you did nothing wrong."

MY JOURNEY

"No matter how far you've gone down the wrong road, you can always turn around." - Turkish Proverb (Author Unknown)

I had been pushed to my breaking point in terms of my professional limits and personal strife by the time Myofascial Release came into my life, long after that conversation with Gram. Physically, I had been dealing with a nagging tightness in my back. Stiff and achy, I started to feel like one of my patients, in constant discomfort. I would alleviate the stiffness by twisting myself in the middle to stretch out the muscles around my spine, but it was a temporary reprieve. Within the hour, I was back at it, struggling to give my body a break.

My head was still full of second-guessing and questions, and my body was hurting when I stepped into my first class. I had done some research and my interest was peaked prior to the speaker's lesson, yet I was not prepared for what he had to say.

I can distinctly remember feeling overwhelmingly let down at first. It seemed to me, an incredible disservice had been done not only to me, but others in my profession. I had never been exposed to fascia the way the speaker presented it. Except for a vague description, in the form of viewing dead and dehydrated fascia on a cadaver in graduate school, we had not been taught exactly what fascia did, or what it could look like in a healthy body. As a physical therapist, how had I not heard about such a crucial component of anatomy, of movement?

The speaker was engaging and spoke on issues that I had found in my patients and been unable to give them lasting relief for. He gave explanations for questions I had filed away in the back of my head for years. Even better, he spoke about back pain that I knew all too well.

He twisted himself into a familiar pose and explained how emotional trauma could cause pain in that area, joking about the way patients would attempt to self-treat it. I had done that exact stretch in my seat only moments before. A wave of realization hit me.

That was only the first (day) of that three day course. By midday of that first class, I noticed something strange. I was sitting at the table, the same as I had when I arrived, however instead of sitting stiffly, my back straight and aching to be twisted and stretched, I sat comfortably. My hands were loose at my sides, my legs uncrossed. I felt free.

In our class on Rebounding, I had explained to the person I was partnered with the day before that I had never unwound before. In fact, I believe I told her, "I simply can't do it." She laughed and confided in me that she hadn't thought she could either.

When we entered the classroom, the lights dimmed and gentle music began to play from the speakers in the front. I would have no choice but to try. We quickly found our treatment table and I scrambled onto it, nervousness creeping up my spine. I laid on my stomach and closed my eyes tight. She began.

I may have thought I couldn't unwind but, as always, my body knew better. She started with a hamstring rebounding technique while I was on my stomach. At first, I resisted and had trouble softening into it. The feeling was preturbing; it is not comfortable to resist rebounding. I realized, lying there, that I was reacting to the memory of being tapped; my body was naturally revolting against the action that I still felt so very annoying. I finally let go and curled up in tears. That was it.

Much later on, I was able to attend the "Therapy for the Therapist" course in Sedona, Arizona. Here, I had the pleasure of being treated three times a day for five days total by therapists who worked directly for John F. Barnes. The therapist that I was assigned to for one of the sessions began by assessing my pelvic alignment. Once she addressed the torsion in my sacrum, she shifted her focus on a different area that had become overtly red while she was working in the pelvic region. She began by putting pressure on my chest. It felt like her other hand was hovering directly over my mouth. I could feel such intense heat in my face. This time, I reacted immediately. I felt my mouth open in a silent scream and very real tears streaming down my face. Heat radiated from every inch of my body and a familiar, hard pit in my stomach began to form.

The movement was different than my last experience on the treatment table. She would not allow me to go through the same, arduous motions from before. At first, I fought the process, struggling to control myself and my emotions. Tears rolled down my face, my throat went desert dry. I sensed that my body had no voice left. I was trying to scream, but nothing was coming out. My body started to tremble. Tremors spread through my extremities, and though I did not yet know it, I began to experience the thawing state of my treatment. My therapist was dialoguing with me and encouraged me to get up, that I could do it, get out from under the hold she was placing on me. She was mirroring the trauma my body had gone through in the past. What I remember from this experience was feeling angry. The sadness was passing and pure anger emerging.

Slowly, my shaking lessened and my twitching ceased. Coldness diffused throughout my flesh into the deepest part of me. Everything came full circle. I was able, at that moment, to let go of all the anger and grief I had held in an iron grasp within my heart. I unwound from all the incomplete cycles I had experienced in my life.

Over the course of that week, I learned many things and brought home many memories that I still think back on fondly. I learned that the concept of unwinding and how to unwind was still very much coming from the analytical, logical, and controlled side of my brain, not from the place that truly mattered.

To truly unwind, you must let go of control, a hard thing for me to do at that point in my life. I realized that during treatment I was trying to evade the compressive techniques in order to retain the control

I thought I needed. They triggered my emotions and memories of the trauma I had experienced during the last night of my old life and part of me resisted that. I had been shoving down the painful memories and emotions for so long, trying to move on with life. I didn't realize how important the extent of that connection was at the time, which is why it is so important to repeat classes.

The beginning of each of my sessions I enjoyed the few minutes that we were given to have a conversation with our therapists. You, of course, can speak at any time during a session in order to convey how you are feeling or ask for them to ease up the pressure on a technique. But, at the beginning it was more in depth, it was a time that we were able to get to know each other and connect. MFR is a deeply emotional therapy and having a form of trust with your practitioner is helpful for both of you.

The therapists I was working with were inquisitive. Questions about my hobbies and personal enjoyment mixed with queries about my family and friends. Their goal was to learn enough about me to tailor my sessions for my needs. I was learning quite a bit too. I was intrigued by their dialoguing skills. The way that they were able to navigate the conversation with skill and grace, gleaning necessary information while respecting the privacy of the patient. I took careful notes. This finesse was perhaps the most important technical skill that I brought home to my own practice. With only a word or two, they were able to strike the exact nerve or emotion that needed to be pushed. Eventually, I honed this key skill as well.

During one such conversation, she asked me when I was going to finally slow down and stop putting so many long hours in at work. She wanted to know when I would begin focusing on starting my own practice. I remember shaking my head and explaining to her the mountains of student loans I had looming over my head and how I had a very aggressive plan to pay it all down before moving on. The strain in my voice as I tried to detail to her the necessity of working 40 hours a week for the outpatient clinic, another 15 hours at the nursing home on weekends, on top of my concierge home visits was painful to hear, even for me.

She was very gentle in asking, when I finally stopped talking, what I was actually scared of. I thought for a moment and answered as plainly as I could: I was afraid that I would fail, that I wouldn't have enough patients to sustain my first year as a full-time clinic, that my passion would not be enough.

There was a moment of silence before she gave a firm pat on the hand. She had once been much like me. Her mentor had asked her the same question that she had and she had given him a similar answer. Now, she wanted to share with me what he had said.

"FEAR stands for False Evidence Appearing Real. The things that seem so utterly terrible now is only your mind coming up with the millions of scenarios that may or may not be true. Sometimes, being fearful is just your subconscious trying to sabotage you. If you want something, go for it."

As I walked out of that last T4T session, I felt a change begin to take place within me. Not only had I achieved a level of calm and peace that I had not thought possible, but my eyes were opened to a new train of thought in regards to patient care, as well as self-treatment. Myofascial Release could be exactly what I had been looking for. Besides the emotional changes, I recognized physical changes, as well; my nagging back pain resolved drastically and my posture greatly improved.

I started to look forward to Mondays again. I challenged myself to use at least two new MFR techniques a day. While every patient requires unique and personalized care, I was able to work pelvic balancing and postural alignment issues into my sessions. I softened my focus and would step back to assess their standing posture from four different perspectives to see where they were holding their tension. Then we would begin with hands on treatment.

My confidence soared as I saw the changes that these new techniques were beginning to make in my patients. They left my office feeling, in their words, different. In my eyes, different was good. I was no longer satiating the immediate need for pain relief, I was finally treating the source.

I could see the causes for a patient's pain or discomfort, not just the symptoms. I knew then this would help them in ways that, before my introduction to MFR, I would have found impossible. Instead of treating the issues I saw in a moment, I was bringing to the present the patient's past, and was able to see a pain-free future.

My bosses were not happy with my newfound treatment. They wanted me on a schedule; one that would be predictable, traditional, and fit within the confines of their comfortable procedures. I was encouraged to begin sessions with a period of modality, having the patient heat or e-stim while I would catch up on my mandatory paperwork. I, instead, chose to jump directly into working one-on-one with patients. This resulted in a large stack of notes to be completed on my desk at the end of the day. For the first time, I did not mind.

I will never forget one of my bosses at the mom-and-pop style outpatient clinic. I was treating a patient with Myofascial Release in one of our shared spaces. She was watching me closely as I closed my eyes and completed the technique. Just before I felt the tissue release fully, her voice reverberated through the room.

"Jessica! Are you sleeping?"

Inside, I was trying to hold it together as best I could, for the patient's sake. I never opened my eyes, but I knew she could see the corners of my mouth curl up into a small smile. I knew that she just didn't understand. This particular boss was carrying around a fair bit of baggage. She wasn't centered, was having issues connecting to patients, and tended to use her patient's physical therapy sessions as talk therapy for herself. I wish she was open to the information I offered; maybe she too, could have found herself in a place of peace.

In my personal life, a change was also beginning to take place. My attitude had shifted and I was more ready with a smile, more open with my feelings; my family and friends could all see it. My goals became larger and my hope ever growing. In fact, I was able to see a future for myself that had been obscured before. I started to make plans to open my own practice.

THE MIND, HEART, AND BODY

"Free your heart from hatred- forgive. Free your mind from worries- most never happen. Live simply and appreciate what you have. Give more. Expect less." - Stephen Covey

Just as I had to realize that change had to come from within myself before I could begin to see progress in my health, patients must become aware that there is more than simple mechanics at work when you enter Myofascial Release treatment. We want to see your mind and body undergo transformation as you become engaged in your therapy and engagement with the emotional aspect of your healing. When you reach this point where both your body and mind can release the blockages that holds them stagnant, you participate in what we call Enlightened Movement.

Let's take it all the way back. I mean, really far. In the early days of the Roman Empire, science and health became the focus of many of the great philosophers at the time. It was then, that our modern understanding of pain and trauma started to take shape. Those ancient philosophers who first advanced the idea that the brain plays a role in producing your perception of pain, drew a connection between how our emotional and mental state played a part in the physical representation of injury and illness in the body. Still, they did not know why.

Fast forward a bit to the 19th century. Physicians and scientists had begun to create a space in Northern Europe that encouraged research and discovery. At the time, progress in medical advancement was all the rage, and we saw the introduction of disease prevention and the beginning stages of antibiotics. We also saw the introduction of opiates in pain relief.

Morphine was found very effective, if addictive, and chemist Felix Hoffman engineered aspirin from a substance in willow bark. Today, both of these methods of pain relief are commonly used. As you can see, the medical field has not progressed much in terms of pain or trauma since then (Academy of Ideas, 2019).

Until 1913, it was widely believed that the psyche was a closed system, meaning that it had no influence on the physical well being of an individual. Swiss psychiatrist, Carl Jung, was studying unconscious awareness and memories at the time and discovered something interesting. Contrary to the popular Fruedian hypothesis of the time, he believed that memories and awareness could be shared by a collective of the same species. He observed this in various insect colonies where survival instinct survived through multiple generations. Insects, even those who were not alive at the time these behaviors were first formed, continued to display them in a consistent manner (Encyclopedia Britannica, 2019).

This was one of the first links between the body and mind that has been studied with practicality. In essence, it is believed that what an individual accepts as their reality becomes just that to them. While Dr. Jung's suppositions opened the door, there was much to uncover about the connection between memory and the mind-body.

Today, we know that this connection manifests itself in the way our body responds to emotional trauma in the past. Our bodies hold emotions in our fascial system like a storage tank, until we are ready to release them. Sometimes, the body holds them in a form we call pain. When you are experiencing MFR, you are peeling away layers of that pain to expose the emotions that are fighting to emerge. Therapists should encourage full expression of all emotions to help your structure release and achieve optimum health.

Walking hand in hand with emotions are the images and memories that may float in and out of your consciousness during or after a treatment. When they surface, they are being released from your tissues. Consider sharing these feelings, as it will aid in your therapist's ability to guide you through your healing process.

Over the course of your treatment your therapist will ask you questions. When answering, allow the response to come from the area of your body being worked on, and not from your head. You do not need to have an understanding of your response or of any emotions that may surface. You always have the option to not answer any question. Never force an answer.

In and out of treatment, I would urge you to listen to the language in which you address yourself. You want to experience life in a positive light, and the easiest way to do that is to be sure that your vocabulary is largely positive. You are a wonder of nature, a creature of beauty; you can achieve all that you wish and more. Tell yourself this, and more, every single chance that you have. Avoid phrases such as, "I can't" or "I never." Keep your mind positive and your body will follow suit.

MISCONCEPTIONS ABOUT MYOFASCIAL RELEASE

*L*ike many cutting edge advances in medicine, Myofascial Release can become misunderstood easily when the public is uninformed. Unlicensed professionals who over simplify the process, or fail to practice the approach directly on skin, and ignorance in general, all play a part in unsubstantiated rumors about what true, authentic Myofascial Release really is. I would like to help expel some of these notions with a quick overview of what is true about Myofascial Release and what is not.

MASSAGE OR
MYOFASCIAL RELEASE

There is some confusion for many as to how Myofascial Release differentiates from massage when an abridged explanation of Myofascial Release is given. While both practices do rely on touch and adjustments to points of fascial restrictions, there are many differences as well. Myofascial Release is, in most cases, very localized and very gentle.

The practitioner performing the therapy should tailor the experience to the unique needs of each and every patient. They should yield to the cues that the patient's body gives and work within the pace that the body sets. Massage, adversely, can be a much more forceful experience and will often push the body past its natural limits, achieving results at the expense of damaged tissue.

You will also notice that there is no sliding or gliding over the surface of your skin during Myofascial Release with the use of oils or lotions. Myofascial Release is performed on dry skin. You will be asked to actively participate in your session as well, whereas with massage you are expected to lie on the table and be worked on mostly in silence; generally people tune out of their body, and may even fall asleep during a massage.

The biggest difference between Myofascial Release and massage is what is happening on the inside. Myofascial Release reaches all the way down to the cellular level, whereas massage only addresses the elastin layer, the superficial 20% surface layer of tissue. Myofascial Release does not push tissue; the main effect is to address inflammation, pain, and motion restrictions, and in order to do this, we want our body's natural anti-inflammatory agent (interleukin 8) to be released.

Rollers and
Other Tools

Some have come to associate Myofascial Release with rolling on foam rollers and other massage tools, which they believe breaks down fascial adhesions, knots, and scar tissue. Though foam rollers are often used in Myofascial Release, when it comes time for self-treatment homework, the issue is with the actual utilization of them.

I often see people at the gym, on television, or even at sporting events aggressively rolling on these tools. This is one of the most frustrating things for me to watch personally, as I know the damage that it does to the tissue. Just seeing the person's grimacing face is enough. When they repetitively roll up and down on the foam roller, they are compressing the free nerve endings that pass through the fascial system, and are creating more damage. Their grimacing face is a sign that they are forcing or bracing the release because rolling over the tool is usually very painful.

I understand the disconnect because the term "rolling" is in the name of the tool. I propose they should rename the tool to "foam releaser," instead of roller. I explain to every patient that I use these tools on the importance of softening into the tissue restrictions and tender points instead of actually rolling. I also stress that you must hold the pressure for an appropriate length of time (three to five minutes or longer) in order for the tissue to soften. Using a foam roller, or other self-treatment tools, is not the same as being treated by an MFR therapist. The cycle of events that we described above from piezoelectricity all the way to resonance does not happen without skin-on-skin contact.

This is because foam rollers do not release fascial restrictions. Their purpose is to help soften them up significantly and assist in maintaining the progress that has been made after a MFR session with a practitioner has taken place.

Another myth pertaining to foam rollers or massage tools is that rolling can help rehydrate the fascial system. In simple terms, our connective tissue is made up of cells, collagen fibers, and a non-living gelatinous matrix called ground substance. When we talk about the fascial system being dehydrated, we are referring to the ground substance of the fascial system.

You cannot restore hydration by just drinking it back into the body. Imagine pouring water over a rock. The rock does not absorb moisture, the water simply rolls away. This is what happens when you try to drink water in an attempt to remedy fascial restrictions. The water doesn't get down to the cellular level, as the restrictions do not allow that level of permeation. After you have Myofascial Release and the spaces in the interstitial web open up, you can drink water and it will permeate through those openings and start to hydrate at the cellular level.

Other tools are even less equipped to deliver on their promise to produce healthier fascia in a user. The name says it all for some. You cannot, and should not, blast or force our fascia into any sort of motion. If you do attempt this, you will only exacerbate any inflammation and pain.

The flaw in the design of these tools is that it forces the tissue to give and that is all. Myofascial Release instead reaches the ground substance within fascia via gentle, sustained compression and stretch. I would not recommend that anyone use this type of device or anything similar. You risk skin discoloration, increased cellulite (though it was originally marketed as a device to decrease cellulite), increase in varicose veins, pain, fatigue, and even weight gain.

WHO NEEDS MFR AND WHY

"If you want different results than what you're getting, you have to try different approaches." - Albert Einstein

I cannot fix you. No therapist can. You may come to me accustomed to lying on other treatment tables, being manipulated and pushed by another individual, hoping that their prodding will find you relief. The only way to heal is for there to be a mutual exchange of understanding and the willingness to do what needs to be done to find the source of the injury. You are your best ally.

Once when I worked in another practice, I overheard an interaction that caused me a great deal of distress. I could hear the patient yelling at her therapist. Her voice was laced with equal parts anger and desperation.

Then, I heard her cry, "Don't you have any compassion?"

Her therapist's response? "Toughen up."

That particular patient suffered from a genetic disorder that put her in chronic pain and exhaustion. She traveled from out of state to receive therapy. My heart hurts for people like her. Even more so because I was once a therapist much like that one. I was hurried, overworked and overbooked, and numb.

It was in that same practice that I had a patient on my schedule that I didn't usually treat. He came in and climbed right down on the table, as he was accustomed to doing with his regular therapist. He had his cell phone in his hands as he lay face down on the table, looking at his phone through the face cradle. I was in awe that this patient expected me to treat him as he responded to emails on his phone. I decided instead to pause and wait for him to realize that our time together was valuable, and not to be used as a work space.

There would not be any multitasking during my session. It took him a few minutes to realize that I hadn't begun the session. When he did, he immediately recognized just how disconnected he had been from therapy. He was so used to getting the "quick fix" by his former therapist, and had lost the mind-body connection that I speak of often to my patients. The rest of the session we addressed his standing alignment and posture before honing in on his pelvic malalignment. The patient learned how to better stay in his body with me. Even though I didn't see him for more than a few sessions, I believe his eyes were opened up to a new way of treatment. When we talk during treatment, we can't fully feel. It is so important to show up and be present.

This patient, and the fact that I did not immediately realize how flawed the system I was working within was, was symptomatic of my personal inconsistencies at that time of my career. My spirit was awoken by my discoveries in Myofascial Release therapy and the way it encourages therapists to treat patients as a whole person, including their mental and emotional state.

In my office, I am quiet when you first meet with me. It is my job to listen, something that fewer and fewer health professionals seem to do. I want you to tell me your story. I want to hear your fears, concerns, and restrictions. Before I touch you, I find out who you are, beyond your symptoms. Too often I am told by my patients, "No one has ever explained it that way to me before. I understand it now."

You may have attempted everything you can imagine, from massage, chiropractic and traditional physical therapy to rolfing, shiatsu, reiki, tai-chi and acupuncture. You may feel as if you have exhausted all choices. Traditional therapies, such as those, rely heavily on labels for diagnosis and treatment. We are conditioned to be symptom focused, and forgo treating the root cause of our health issues in favor of subduing the immediate discomfort. Similarly, in traditional physical therapy clinics, because they are largely run by insurance companies, therapists are often restricted by times dictated by units and reimbursements. In turn, patients get the "quick fix" approach, and therapists burn out from having to treat more patients a day.

THE FASCIAL PELVIS

"Over 90 % of patients suffering with lumbar and pelvic pain, menstrual problems, cervical pain, and headaches have imbalances in the pelvis creating fascial restrictions throughout the body." John F. Barnes, PT

The word "pelvis" originates from the Latin word for "basin." This is a fitting term, as a basin's most basic function is to hold fluids. Trauma and inflammatory responses tend to dehydrate ground substance within the fascial system, an issue for organisms like you and I, who are 70% fluid. In other words, when our basin runs dry, we begin to experience pain.

You may be surprised that pelvic health is important in both men and women and can be treated in similar ways. Due to the nature of the pelvic floor, the way that the layers of muscle are surrounded by fascia, a balance of stability in relation to mobility is needed for it to function properly. It needs to be pliable in order to allow for expulsion, as well as flexible for reproductive functions. The muscle tone should be adequate in order to provide stability, while not sacrificing the elasticity.

A therapist can assess if deficiency in either is the cause of unexplained pain by determining if the patient requires stretching and relaxation in order to maximize mobility, or if strengthening of the muscle to promote support is needed. The true goal of treatment should focus on balancing the pelvis in order to create stability for the rest of the skeletal structure.

Keeping this in mind, let's imagine that a patient is complaining of pain radiating from internal organs, such as the stomach or bladder, with no discernible cause. Traditional therapies may write it off and the patient could be prescribed pain medication as a temporary fix.

Instead, I propose that there could be an abdominal scar from a cesarean section surgery that is putting pressure on the bladder and contributing to lumbar back pain, or hypertonus or trigger points in the abdominal muscles that has manifested itself in the pelvic area. It could also be piriformis syndrome, wherein the sciatic nerve and obturator internus form a sandwich and a sciatic nerve is being impinged upon; usually they all stem back to pelvic imbalance as the origin. These issues can be treated effectively with Myofascial Release Therapy.

In a more extreme example, let's say that a patient is experiencing painful intercourse, impotence, or incontinence. They could also have some discomfort while sitting. They could very well be suffering from pudendal nerve entrapment, which is a type of chronic pelvic pain caused by the compression of the pudendal nerve due to tightened fascia, muscles, or internal adhesions.

Our bodies are covered in nerve receptors. Certain areas have many more than the rest. The autonomic, lumbosacral nerve plexus is one such cluster in your gut. Some actually refer to the gut as your second brain due to this fact. It provides hammock-like support for organs in the pelvic diaphragm, such as the intestines. 90% of the body's serotonin and 50% of dopamine are made in this area, as well. If fascia is restricted, it won't just affect the vertebra (lumbar/sacrum/discs), it can also affect the function of our organs, causing problems with urination, bowel function, and digestion (Courses.lumenlearning.com, 2019).

By providing gentle, sustained, hands-on compression and stretch into the areas of fascial restriction, a MFR therapist can restore the necessary slack to the system to take the pressure off of the pudendal nerve and surrounding structures that may be far away from the pelvic region. This helps to eliminate pain and improve the ability to sit, engage in intercourse, and maintain continence.

Pudendal Nerve Entrapment (PNE)

Also known as Alcock canal syndrome, PNE occurs when the pudendal nerve (which is located in the pelvis) becomes entrapped or compressed. This pain is worsened by sitting and other positions that involve the compression of the pelvis. PNE is a common side effect of repetitive exercises like biking, as well as a sedentary lifestyle. It can happen when you're injured, have surgery, or give birth. This can affect both men and women.

Symptoms:
- Aches and pains
- Shooting pains down the leg
- Difficulty moving/stretching your pelvic region
- A frequent need to go to the bathroom
- Pain during sex

PELVIC NERVE ENTRAPMENT

*N*erve entrapment is a condition that can happen throughout our bodies as a result of repetitive injuries we incur over time. In men, it is common to cause these injuries to the pelvic muscles specifically at work in laborious jobs, lifting, working out, and aging. Each of these can kick start the "trapping of nerves" in the general region. Accidents such as fractures, broken bones, and frequent sprains can all cause nerve compression syndrome as well.

Symptoms:
- Aches and pains
- Inflammation
- Tingling or numbness
- Reduced flexibility
- Difficulty moving/stretching your pelvic region

MARIA'S STORY

*M*aria has been a patient at Arancia since the summer of 2019. She called the clinic looking for guidance regarding pelvic health matters. Having already tried pelvic health physical therapy at another location, she was nervous and skeptical, rightfully so. She explained she was considering a trial at a clinic that was closer to her home, but it did not practice Women's Health specific Myofascial Release. I did what I do with everyone who calls my clinic, I listened to her unique story.

As she spoke, I so badly wanted to interject, and tell her, "I know I can help, you did the right thing by calling. Let's get started!" I sometimes have to put my hand over my mouth, to keep from doing that too soon, because what I often hear from my patients is that no one has taken the time to really listen fully to their story.

This is a core value at Arancia. We listen, we want to truly get to know you first, hear your full story, then make 100% sure we are a good fit for you. If we are not a good fit, we strive to place you somewhere that will be.

When Maria had reached the end of her story, I asked her a few questions and gave her another opportunity to share with me. I was able to share at that point that I have treated patients just like her, and that she is not crazy. Instead, I told her that she was very intelligent and intuitive for being so in tune with her body and what she is feeling, which is a characteristic that not many people possess.

After our first conversation, Maria decided to come to Arancia for a complimentary discovery visit. I believe people should be allowed to come into the clinic and get a good sense of whether or not we are a good fit for them. I want their nerves and skepticism to ease, and feel confident with the decision to start therapy under my care.

At the end of her discovery visit, Maria decided to sign up for an evaluation, the only catch was that soon after that evaluation, she was off to Hawaii for a vacation with her husband. She was very eager to start therapy with the hopes of getting relief before having to sit on a plane for over 11 hours each way.

I was a little concerned with her expectations and explained that although she may feel less tension and more ease in her body, things get a bit stirred up before getting better, although it varies across the board. Maria came back after her trip and was excited and eager to tell me that she managed well on the plane, and didn't have any new upsets. We set up a plan of care based on my evaluation findings and Maria's goals, and we began treatments.

Maria has been by far one of the most compliant and devoted patients I have had the pleasure of knowing. She truly understands the importance of mind and body connection, and knows that she will need to place emphasis on self-treatment and regular treatment "tune-ups" for life. She is not unique in that sense. We should all be getting treated on a regular basis, even if we are not in pain.

The best part about this is that she needs me much less now, as she is able to identify what to do when she is feeling her tissue restrictions. She listens carefully to her body and self-treats regularly. She is empowered. Prevention is the key to aging gracefully!

From Maria

"I am happy that I suffer from Pudendal Neuralgia. Happy because I now have a diagnosis for what had significantly impacted my life for more than three months and was getting more painful and debilitating each and every day. The journey to obtaining this diagnosis was excruciatingly slow, frustrating, and exhausting, both physically and mentally.

It could very well have gone on for numerous months, if not years, had I not been so determined to end my pain. Not knowing what is causing your pain makes it very difficult and frustrating to treat. When numerous medical professionals are also perplexed as to what is causing your pain, you begin to question yourself and lose hope. With a diagnosis, you can then explore treatment options. Myofascial Release Therapy has altered the trajectory of my life, the quality of my life, and the outlook of my life. I wish to share my story in the hope that your story is much shorter than mine. I also want you to see the benefits of perseverance, to never lose your voice or your hope!

My story begins with me having discomfort while sitting. When I sat, I could no longer tolerate the pressure of my pants touching my vaginal area. I had to get up frequently as the irritation was constant, increasing, and very distracting. I had not gained weight and my pants were not tight. When I stood I felt some relief, but not complete relief. I made an appointment with my OBGYN and a small cyst on the outside of my vagina was discovered and removed. What I hoped to be the end of my discomfort was not; unfortunately, it was only the beginning. The irritation seemed to disappear, but returned a week or so later. I returned to my OBGYN and told them I knew my body and things just weren't right down there. They concluded I had an external yeast infection, even though I did not present with typical symptoms. I was given a topical steroid to apply. I was subsequently treated for an internal yeast infection, and then three weeks later, a urinary tract infection.

In hindsight, I don't think I really ever had a yeast infection to begin with and believe the treatment for the yeast infection led to a UTI, which compounded my symptoms. I was calling and going to the OBGYN on a weekly basis for almost 10 weeks in an attempt to seek treatment for the burning feeling I was constantly having. At first I could not sit because of the burning, then I had burning when standing, as well as when I wiped after urinating and defecating. I was told to "wipe gently." I was also told the excruciating pain, burning, and sometimes numbness I was now experiencing in my groin 'was not' related to the burning in my vaginal area. A CAT scan of my pelvis revealed nothing.

I believe my OBGYN was doing their best to help me, but the process as a patient was incredibly frustrating. I simply did not feel as though I was being heard or believed during this process. I felt marginalized. Out of sheer desperation and so much distress both physically and mentally, I would sometimes merely show up at their office, seeking help. I felt the staff just looked at me like I was some crazy woman. My visits were so frequent that it got to the point I didn't even have to give my name, the entire staff knew it and it was a large staff. I kept telling them I knew my body and something was very wrong. I have since learned Pudendal Neuralgia does not show up on X-rays, CAT scans, or even MRIs. The pudendal nerve runs from the anus through the vagina and groin. Stress exacerbates the symptoms of PN. The arduous process I was on to seek a diagnosis and resolution of my symptoms, unknowingly, was significantly compounding my symptoms.

To my dismay, my OBGYN said they had exhausted all options and I should consider trying a Pelvic Pain Center. Getting an appointment would take months and I could not wait months; I could barely make it through a day. No longer able to work, sit, walk, lie down or drive, I went to my primary care doctor. He did not think it was an issue with a hernia I had repaired many years ago. He felt it was an inflammation and prescribed me an anti-inflammatory medicine. A hip X-ray revealed nothing. The medicine lessened my symptoms somewhat, but I still ended up returning to my primary care doctor for additional visits and the ER twice due to the debilitating pain.

The cause of my distress was still undetermined, so I saw a general surgeon to confirm it was not hernia related. It was confirmed it was not hernia related and he suggested I see an Orthopedic Specialist. The Orthopedic Specialist was equally baffled by my symptoms, as the X-ray and MRI he ordered on my pelvis revealed nothing. He was very sympathetic to my plight and my long journey and agreed to help me, even if it appeared it was not in his area of expertise. He prescribed nerve medicine, as he thought it might be nerve related. His recommendation was to go back to my OBGYN or go to a pain clinic. Since my back was now hurting due to my inability to sit and walk properly, I asked him to authorize me to see a physical therapist. During the three week wait to get an appointment, I was feeling better while taking the nerve and anti-inflammatory medicine. I could sit and walk a bit better.

Within five minutes of meeting with a physical therapist and describing my symptoms, she stated she felt I was suffering from Pudendal Neuralgia. Wait! A diagnosis! After all I have been through! Regrettably, our visit ended as quickly as it started, as she said she was not trained to help me with this issue. I needed to see a physical therapist trained in the pelvic floor area. With her help, I secured an appointment with an appropriate PT. I shudder to wonder where I would be today had I not suggested getting authorization to see a physical therapist.

I felt this PT was my savior. After two and a half months of twice a week traditional physical therapy, I was able to sit and walk with little to no discomfort. I had never been to PT before so I did not know what to expect. Although the true cause of Pudendal Neuralgia isn't known, my PT felt it may have resulted from the scar tissue from the cyst I had removed months before. I informed her I had previously had a hernia removed in the very spot on the side of my groin that was extremely painful. The bulk of the PT consisted of external massages in the groin and pelvic area. I was given daily stretching exercises to do on my own. A handful of times she did a rectum or vaginal release. To be fair, by the time I found her, my pelvic area was so tight it took many visits before she could do anything internally. She also gave me relaxation techniques to incorporate into my day. I continually asked if my improvement was due to the medicine I had just started taking or the PT, and she said a combination of both. Since I do not like taking medicine of any kind, I was eager to get off of them as soon as possible. I also wanted my routine back, my life back, after seven months of hell. When I could sit and walk burning and pain-free, I started reducing my medicine and ended PT. She was supportive of my request and felt I had made tremendous progress. I thought I was cured, and this nightmare was behind me. Regrettably, six weeks after I stopped taking medicine and ending PT, on a quiet, Friday afternoon, I felt that dreadful burning feeling start up again.

I tried not to believe it was back. I tried to fight it off, dismiss it, suck it up, but after a month I had to surrender and get back on the medicine, as the burning and pain were too debilitating to ignore. It had come back with a vengeance. I had to gradually increase the dosage to a greater dosage than I had ever been on before. Not only was I devastated at its return, I felt defeated. I was confident my issue with Pudendal Neuralgia was put to rest. It was not. Even with ever increasing dosages of medicine, I was still unable to sit once again. I had religiously continued doing the self-care exercises my PT had prescribed. My office desk was converted to a sit/stand set up so I could continue to work. I did not want to take more medicine or take medicine for the rest of my life. I truly wanted to get to the root of why I had PN. Through extensive research on my part, which by the way, was easier this time since I now had a diagnosis, I learned about Myofascial Release Therapy. MFR is a therapy that treats chronic pain caused by trauma, scarring, and inflammation by releasing tension in the myofascial tissue throughout your body. I was intrigued.

As you can imagine, I was also skeptical of yet another physical therapy practice. I had just committed close to three months of twice weekly sessions, and despite my earnest commitment, PN returned. I found a Myofascial Release Therapist who was also a certified Physical Therapist in my area and contacted her. After sharing my long and arduous journey thus far with her, she was confident Myofascial Release Therapy could help me. I had to make a decision. I could return to my prior PT, who did help me sit and walk while taking medicine, or I could try Myofascial Release Therapy, with the hope that we can get to the root of the burning/pain and eventually get off medicine all together. My first PT was covered in full under my insurance, whereas this new PT does not take insurance and would come with a hefty out-of-pocket expense.

I had followed my gut my entire journey, and it told me to give Dr. Jessica Papa, owner of Arancia Physical Therapy, a try. Dr. Jess is a certified Physical Therapist, as well as an Expert Level Myofascial Release Therapist. From the onset, Dr. Jess was confident Myofascial Release Therapy could help me, especially when she saw my 24 year old cesarean scar, and took note of a hernia surgery on the very side of my groin that was also causing me tremendous pain. Dr. Jess informed me scar tissue can significantly restrict the structure and function of myofascial tissue. With restriction comes burning and pain. This was a logical explanation of why I had PN. My scar from the cyst removal was external, yet the scars from my cesarean section and hernia were very deep and decades old. None of the numerous medical professionals I saw on my journey for relief ever connected these two scars and their close proximity to my areas of discomfort, pelvic and right groin, except for Dr. Jess. My heart and gut told me these scars had significantly contributed to my PN. I now think the shingles I had years ago in the lower pelvic area, which resulted in nerve damage, is also a contributor. I have since learned from my sessions with Dr. Jess that stress can exacerbate myofascial restrictions. I have been battling Irritable Bowel Syndrome for the last 30 years, which no doubt has increased my daily level of stress. It sounded like Myofascial Release Therapy could help improve many aspects of my life.

I began my treatment with Dr. Jess by going to twice a week sessions. This PT experience is completely different than my prior sessions with a traditional PT. Depending upon my complaint area of the day, it would dictate what treatment the session would consist of. Due to the nature of PN, most of the sessions for me consist of internal releases within the vagina and anus. You need to leave your modesty at the door. You work as a team with Dr. Jessica. While treating you, she will ask you to describe in detail what you are feeling at that moment. At first I would say, "feeling good." I soon learned she wanted to hear if I felt burning, pulling, pain, pulsating, warmth, etc. My response would then guide her to either reduce the pressure, extend the release, etc. Little did I know it was also her way to help me to dial into my body. For me to get a deeper understanding of how it works, interpret what I was feeling, and what my body was asking for. This dialogue has become invaluable when I do my daily self-care at home. If I feel warmth, I know a release is occurring. If I feel the pain, I know to reduce the pressure, but extend the release time in that area a bit longer.

I have learned that Myofascial Release Therapy will not be a quick fix for me. My restrictions probably started decades ago, so it is very unrealistic to think that I can un-do and retrain how my myofascial tissue should work in weeks or months. I am pleased that in less than three months of treatment with Dr. Jess, I have been able to reduce my medicine, as well as the frequency of my sessions with her. I have my life back. I can work, walk, sit, lie down, bike, ski, travel, and enjoy life again. I have learned that long-term success with Myofascial Release Therapy requires a lifestyle change. You must commit to a daily self-treatment plan. I absolutely love learning how I can help myself and treat myself.

Without a doubt, having PN is very challenging! Becoming aware of Myofascial Release Therapy has empowered me and made me believe I can significantly influence its impact on my life. I am incredibly grateful that I now have the knowledge and the self-care techniques to treat myself. Since PN is impacted by your emotions, breathing, stress levels, diet, digestion, posture and weather, how you feel during the day is very variable. Learning how to decipher what you feel, why you feel it, and then having the knowledge/techniques to bring about change is incredible and powerful. If you pay attention, you CAN change how you feel and prevent your pain from escalating. I am still a work in progress with this process.

Myofascial Release Therapy and Dr. Jessica Papa have forever changed my life. I believe it can change your life if you give it a chance. I chose to share my story in Dr. Jessica's book because we both agree my journey to finding and learning about the benefits of Myofascial Release Therapy should not have been as long or be as difficult. If I can shorten your story or lessen your pain, then even more benefits have come from my struggles. I do not fault the medical professionals I encountered on my journey. They did their best with what they knew. I did write to them and inform them that my "mystery pain" is probably Pudendal Neuralgia and related to scar tissue from decades ago. Hopefully when they encounter another patient like me, suffering from similar symptoms, they will remember me, and refer them to a physical therapist who is trained in John F. Barnes Myofascial Release Therapy. I know my body, and Myofascial Release Therapy works for me! I feel we all have an obligation to pay things forward."

WOMEN'S HEALTH

*T*he unique way that women's bodies are designed can lend itself to unique pain that modern medicine is still attempting to address. As we explored previously, women make up a large demographic of my clientele. From complications associated with pregnancy, postpartum, unexplained pelvic pain, prolapse, infertility to menstrual discomfort, female patients can find that many of their unexplained pains can be treated effectively with Myofascial Release Therapy. I personally treat all of the above, as well as adhesions, coccygeal pain, dysmenorrhea (painful menstruation), dyspareunia (painful intercourse), endometriosis, infertility, interstitial cystitis, pelvic floor dysfunction, urinary incontinence, urgency, frequency, vulvodynia and breast pain, pre and post-mastectomy on a regular basis.

First, let's explore the issues that can be present due to issues within the pelvic area. The pelvic cavity contains all reproductive organs, the bladder, pelvic colon, and rectum, surrounded by pelvic bones. Each of these components work together and affect one another, both in function and accessibility. When one is changed or moved due to surgery or pregnancy, another compensates in return.

The pelvic floor serves as the base for all of this, a muscular plate that is constantly working to support all of these organs against the downward forces of intra-abdominal pressure. As with the rest of your tissue, it is also completely enveloped in fascia, and in so, can be treated with Myofascial Release Therapy. It acts as a sling to support the bladder, uterus, and rectum, specifically. These deep muscles are connected to the tailbone, sacrum, and hip bones, securely surrounding the urethra and vulva. Because of this strategic placement, it assists in important functions, such as urination and defecation. This portion of the anatomy needs to be strong and healthy, while retaining flexibility to accommodate the movement needed for bowel movements, urination, and childbirth.

Above the pelvic cavity is the abdominal core. Imagine, if you will, a box. Think of the diaphragm as the top, the pelvic floor as the bottom, and the deepest abdominal muscle, the transversus abdominus, as the sides, wrapping around the entirety of the box, making up the portion that supports the top while protecting the bottom. Within this box is where intra-abdominal pressure is generated. You can feel the sensation of this pressure being developed when you sneeze or cough. To counteract this generous pressure, we need to be sure that our pelvic fascia is healthy and working the way that it should.

On top of all this, it is imperative that as a woman, you are tracking pain and discomfort throughout your body, as it could very well stem from unseen issues in the pelvic region. I have had many patients who come in complaining of aching and sharp pain in their back with no apparent cause. They are often surprised when I suggest that this pain may be stemming from the pelvic floor. More often than not, these cases of unexplained pain are present in women who have given birth or had a hysterectomy. The fascial restrictions resulting from trauma related to these events can place an excessive amount of pressure on the organs and result in pelvic organ prolapse. We see here, in action, the domino effect: one portion of the body affecting the next until the origin is lost in the chaos of pain.

All of these muscles coordinate, working together, to control this pressure when it arises. This is done to assist in stabilizing the abdominopelvic organs and help support the lower back. Once you understand how each cog in the machine works with one another, you can see why it is imperative to consider all of the muscles associated with the abdominal core when there is an issue within the pelvic floor, rather than focusing purely on the pelvic floor when looking to treat the source of pain, as many traditional therapies do.

INFERTILITY, PREGNANCY AND BIRTH

*U*nexplained infertility is on the rise. I have had many women who have gone through rounds of fertility treatments, and given up the idea of conceiving a child naturally, come into my office to be treated for unrelated pain. Through regular treatments, there have been cases in which the patients have become pregnant. I attribute this to the whole-body healing that MFR treatments can have.

Let's say we have a patient who has chosen to try MFR therapy strictly to treat their infertility. Our first step is to perform a thorough posture assessment before beginning treatment. This analysis gives the therapist a good idea of where the tissue is pulling from and how it is affecting the fascia throughout the whole body. Since symptoms can be far from the place where the injury originated, if an injury is involved, the therapist should always ask for a thorough medical history. Often, the restrictions that are causing the infertility can be treated as long as the therapist is aware that it is there.

A common cause for infertility that has been deemed unexplained is adhesions in the pelvic region. Because of the fact that these adhesions are invisible to medical imaging, it has become a mysterious, frustratingly untreatable condition. Through treatments, the aim is to release these invisible adhesions in order to trigger a decrease in tissue restrictions around reproductive organs. I am so glad to say that I have seen pregnancies achieved in such cases and normal reproductive function restored.

Mystery around Women's Health issues extend past infertility, of course. Endometriosis, while a common cause of infertility, also affects women who are not attempting to conceive. It is inflammation located in the lining of the uterine cavity, causing tissue to grow outside of the uterus. Endometriosis is linked to extremely painful and heavy menstrual cycles. Traditional medicine is limited in the treatment of this disorder because of the difficulty diagnosing it, and being unable to treat it long-term without affecting fertility. MFR has found great success in women who have endometriosis by decreasing tightness and fascial restrictions around the pelvis, effectively lessening the patient's inflammation, and ultimately, her pain.

Let's say you are a part of the nearly 50% of women who give birth at least once in their life. For most, birth can be an incredibly traumatic event. Episiotomy scars can cause pain and tightness in the area; a broken coccyx, or tailbone, can occur, and if you happen to have a cesarean section, surgery can lead to long-term issues with fascia. When I talk about broken tailbones in laboring women, I get a lot of winces in response, surprisingly just as often as when I speak about the other, more well-known risks. I believe this is because you don't necessarily consider the amount of pressure that is put on the coccyx during birth. Most often, the injury occurs because the tailbone is displaced anteriorly during a long or particularly intense labor and delivery. It can also be extended too far back or pulled off to either side. Because the pelvic floor muscles attach to the tailbone, a change in its position can also change the length and tension of the muscles, thus affecting their tone and strength. As a result, incontinence and pelvic problems or pain can occur. Yes, let's all say it together, ouch!

The pressure that is put on the body during labor and birth far exceeds the expectations anybody can have of their pain threshold. At the point of a baby being born, quite a bit of trauma occurs, and some symptoms present themselves as postpartum depression. Seeking therapy is beneficial to a new mother, physically and emotionally. Treatment can include balancing the pelvis, opening your spine, and releasing the occipital condyle area. MFR for the cranial area can be extremely calming and therapeutic.

It is so important for women to be treated before, during, and after pregnancy. For various reasons, such as weight gain causing the pelvis to tilt anteriorly, joint laxity, sciatica, ligament strain, back pain, diastasis recti, carrying a baby on your hip causing muscular imbalances, or wearing high heels, our pelvis can become misaligned, creating uneven forces on the rest of our body. Our body can only compensate for so long until we start to feel the ramifications of those compensations. When your center of gravity, which starts at S2 (your second sacral segment), is off nothing else in the body can line up evenly. So over time, the problem that started at the pelvis, can reach all the way up to the skull, causing headaches, hip pain, sacral pain, back pain, knee pain, and more.

As a woman, one of the scarier issues that can arise is pelvic organ prolapse. This is when the muscles, ligaments, and connective tissues become weak and the organs descend. Women who experience this may have pain associated with their back, pressure in the abdominal area, and feel as if their groin is going to come completely off. Additionally, they may not be able to have intercourse without some amount of discomfort.

Uterine prolapse is one of the more common types of pelvic organ prolapse, and one that I see often. The uterus, in women who suffer from this, descends into the vaginal wall creating a noticeable bulge within the vagina. In patients who have undergone a hysterectomy, the very top of the vagina can descend into the lower half instead. If the descent of the uterus or vagina is not complete, the issue can oftentimes be addressed by implementing a stabilization program that has been designed to help the uterus lift and provide support. In the case that the organs have descended past the point of natural recovery, mesh or a sling can be placed to lend support.

As important as birth and pregnancy is, the pelvis has another important function that we never want to ignore: intercourse. Dyspareunia is the medical term for pain before, during, and after intercourse. It may affect 20-50% of women (Seehusen, Baird and Bode, 2019). The causes range from physical to emotional trauma. The treatment for dyspareunia is restricted. Many women do not feel comfortable sharing with their medical provider that they are struggling with it, and even worse, besides muscle relaxants and talk therapy, there is not much to be done. With MFR, a therapist can help you find release, helping to relax fascial restrictions, and eventually treating the cause of the disorder.

Pain should not be hidden behind a cloud of mystery. We want to confront it head on so that you can move through life with your head and heart held high. As a woman, everything from sex to birth to monthly menstration can be a source of discomfort; let us come together with information and understanding to bring the issues that affect so many of us to the light, so that we can treat it in the best possible way we know how.

INCONTINENCE

*D*o you have a hard time holding your bladder, even long enough to make it to the toilet? What about having trouble controlling your bowels? If you experience leakage when you sneeze, laugh, or exercise, or have issues with passing gas, there is a great chance that you can be diagnosed with stress incontinence. In women, bladder problems, including incontinence, affects over 30% of women in their 30s, and over 60% of women over 50. So, if you are struggling, you are in good company.

Let's start with the basics. Your bladder expands as urine begins to fill it. Normally, valve-like muscles in the urethra, the tube that transports urine from your body, is closed during the time. This prevents the urine from leaking until you reach a bathroom and relax those muscles. The issue of incontinence occurs when those muscles weaken and are unable to withstand the pressure abdominal and pelvic muscles exert when in motion. If you suffer from stress incontinence, you will be unable to hold your urine when your organs are under this pressure, such as when you laugh or sneeze.

A secondary type of incontinence can be referred to as urge incontinence. In contrast with losing control of your bladder due to pressure, when you suffer from this type, unwilling urination can occur without stimuli. If you get the urge to empty your bladder, there should be a time period in which you can hold it in order to make the trip to an appropriate place to do so. If you cannot and your bladder contracts involuntarily, causing leakage, you just might be feeling the affects of this affliction. To combat this, a physical therapist specializing in pelvic health may work with you on fascial restrictions, bladder retraining, and alignment. They may also suggest bladder releases.

There are many factors that contribute to an individual experiencing incontinence, age being the most common. Although stress incontinence isn't a normal part of the physical changes associated with aging, it can make you more susceptible due to the general weakening of the muscles. It is expected that a person who has reached an older age will have small bouts of incontinence. This can be treated effectively with pelvic physical therapy.

Delivery of a child also can be a factor in developing incontinence. Women who have had a vaginal delivery are more likely to develop urinary incontinence than a woman who has given birth via cesarean section. However, c-section scars can contribute to increased fascial pressure placed upon the organs to include the bladder. On top of this, women whose deliveries have also included the use of forceps have the greatest risk of stress incontinence.

The third consideration is body weight. People, especially women, who are overweight or obese, have a much higher risk of incontinence than those at a healthy weight. This is because excessive weight puts pressure on the abdominal and pelvic organs. If the pelvic floor is not equipped to handle this extra pressure, leakage can occur.

Lastly, if you have had previous pelvic surgery, such as a hysterectomy, incontinence can become an issue. The bladder and urethra's functions can be altered by the actual procedure or the scarring that occurs when healed. Ligaments and other tissues can be affected, dropping your organs down. Patients who suffer from incontinence because of this will often find themselves feeling the effects long after the typical recovery period.

Bladder issues are relieved with MFR because MFR treatments can decrease the tightness and spasms in the pelvic floor muscles and the tissues surrounding the bladder. Not addressing this tightness can lead to urgency, frequency issues, overactive bladder, and leakage, so it is imperative to seek out treatment as soon as possible.

Although all of this can be expected, it is not a reason to go out and buy a package of Depends just yet. There are treatment options for each subtype of person who might be dealing with incontinence, and furthermore, exercises that can help prevent incontinence at later stages of your life.

When seeking treatment, there are a few techniques you can practice at home. First, when urinating, be sure to keep the pelvic floor fully relaxed and allow for opening of the sphincters and urine to flow freely. Resist any urge to use your muscles to push the urine out quickly or forcefully. There are two reasons for this. One, you will have unrelaxed pelvic floor musculature, and two, you have put an increased amount of pressure on the pelvic floor that can result in pelvic organ prolapse.

Do not allow your bladder to fill to capacity. Try to be aware of your body and listen to earlier cues that may indicate that you need to go. In that same vein of thought, always urinate before leaving on a long trip or going somewhere that may not have access to restrooms. In addition, be sure to clean yourself thoroughly after every visit to the restroom. Do not rush. Leaving residue behind will lead to an increased frequency of urination, and ultimately, urinary tract infections. Infections can then, in turn, cause a worsening of leakage.

Incontinence does not only refer to urinary issues. Bowel incontinence can also become an issue for a myriad of reasons. One such reason could be constipation. To combat this, it is important to be aware of your posture when defecating. A normal anorectal angle is around 80-100 degrees. Now, when you squat while on the toilet using a step stool or another, similar device, you can create an even greater angle. The better the angle, the greater ease of transit.

Making it easier for you to go is important because naturally occurring reflexes are more effective than those produced by bearing down. So, to combat constipation, start paying attention to your gastrocolic reflex, the psychological signal to your brain that informs your bowels that it is time to go based on subconscious cues.

For most people the gastrocolic reflex is most active in the morning, just after you wake up, and immediately after a meal. I recommend that patients who are dealing with this particular issue, sit on the toilet after breakfast every day, even when they do not feel the urge to go. This can assist in training your reflex to associate that time of day with defecating. If you can treat the cause of bowel incontinence, in this case constipation, you have treated your body as a whole and not only fixed the issue, but prevented it from returning.

Avoiding common bladder irritants can be helpful, as well. Many people do not realize that carbonation, such as seltzer and soda pop, can wreak havoc on the bladder. Caffeine, processed foods, artificial sweeteners, alcohol, tea, chocolate, spicy food, and citrus are also not great for the gut. While most people do not need to lower their intake of drinks that contain carbonation, I do recommend it to patients that suffer from incontinence as a first line of defense.

On top of all of this, it is imperative to strive for a generally healthy digestive system. This includes eating healthy and being sure to take in the proper amount of fiber every day to keep everything else you eat moving through your system. Women under 50 years old need at least 25 grams of fiber, while men need 38 grams. The recommendation does decrease when a patient has reached the age of 50.

I see patients on a regular basis about other bladder conditions as well, that may or may not result in incontinence. One of the more common issues is called Interstitial Cystitis. This condition is characterized by urinary frequency, urgency, and pressure and pain on the bladder or pelvis. Though there is no known cause, it has been suggested that it may be linked to trauma at an early age, causing emotional distress and inflammation (Seehusen, Baird and Bode, 2019).

BREAST HEALTH

*M*any gynecologists tell patients to familiarize themselves with their breasts by checking them monthly and noting changes in size, shape and skin texture, as well as checking for discharge, rashes, or lumps. When you are self-checking your breasts, you are assessing the quality and texture of your tissue. You want to feel for anything that is hot, hard or tender, or that can signify a fascial/connective tissue restriction. Go slow and be gentle. Compare both sides.

TREAT YOUR BREASTS:

*I*f you do feel a spot that is hot, hard or tender, and unlike the rest of the breast tissue, don't panic. First, gently apply light pressure into the area, holding for a minimum of three to five minutes. Remember, you don't want to force the tissue, or massage it. Gently compress into the hard or tender spot and soften into it. Aim to self-treat your breasts at least two times a week for five minutes or longer. If the area doesn't soften, be sure to address it with your doctor.

SURGERY

*M*ost people are aware of the positive aspects of surgery. A surgeon can perform a total knee replacement, transplant a kidney or heart, repair fractured bones, and suture wounds caused by an accident. This is indisputably good.

The problem is that the more advanced surgery gets, the more it is mistaken with "treatment of choice," instead of the "last resort." From what I have observed, most people do not understand the implication of cutting and surgically altering the body. The truth is, our body is not a car and parts can't be made in a factory and swapped in at the nearest body shop.

In reality, the body is much better off without surgery, if it can be avoided. This applies to plastic surgery as well. I have had countless patients whose augmentations range from nips and tucks here and there, to major plastic surgery procedures, including face lifts, breast implants and back sculpting, as well as liposuction. Lets face it, they are all seeing me because of the limitations that surgery, scar tissue, and adhesions have created, often far from the incision sites. Surgery should be seen as a vital part of emergency care as opposed to a solution or treatment of preventable diseases.

It is vital to know that in many cases the cause of the problem, such as disc prolapse, chronic disease, or cancer, often lies elsewhere. My mentor always explains that the word "disease" stands for "lack of ease" within the body. Breaking it down: dis (lack of) ease, lack of ease. That can contribute to altered movement patterns, repetitive movements, inflammation, and more.

This year, thousands of women in the United States diagnosed with breast cancer will undergo the removal of breast tissue, a procedure called a mastectomy. Though not widely known, it is imperative that you seek treatment for the scars that you will receive because of this surgery, as it is for all scarring. (American Cancer Society, 2017)

The very first thing that the scalpel cuts into with any surgery is the connective tissue, aka your fascial system. Fascia lays over muscle and goes all the way down to the cellular level. This is where inflammation begins and brews. If scars are left untreated, they can develop adhesions, which will continue to dehydrate the fascial system, ultimately affecting surrounding areas, causing neck, shoulder, head, even jaw issues.

SCARRING

So far we have talked a great deal about how pain can come from unseen sources. While this is true very often, we must also take into account a very visible source of fascial disruption: scarring. Unlike a weak pelvic floor or emotional trauma, scars are a mark of a physical event that can clearly tell us where the pain is originating.

You might be wondering why someone would choose to undergo MFR treatments when scarring indicates healing by its very nature. Scars can be tricky. They are usually external, meaning you can see the damage that has been done to your skin from the outside. What you cannot discern from a scar is the extent of the damage that was caused at deeper levels. Damaging your tissue disrupts fibrillar harmony, no matter how small of an injury you sustain. As such, you can expect to experience symptoms long after the injury seems to be healed.

Adhesions are the real culprit when it comes to being sure that a scarred area is left healthy. When you are cut for any reason, the physiological mechanisms your body has to combat the trauma is to seal the wound quickly and efficiently, eventually producing a scar. Adhesions are an internal complication that goes hand in hand with this process. It is present in simple instances of cuts, as well as in the presence of inflammatory diseases or conditions, such as complex regional pain syndrome. They can spread out from the scar site throughout the body like vines, reaching places that you are not even aware are connected.

Because they create soft tissue restrictions far from the original, visible scar, they can lead to concerning symptoms that include pain, sensitivity, numbness, tingling, and dense build up of tissue. The good news is that, unlike scars, adhesions are susceptible to manual change. When treated by a therapist who specializes in MFR, you can see softening and returned flexibility in the tissue because they are able to help your body achieve healing within the fascia. As such, the symptoms and pain that have been caused by these adhesions lessen, or eventually, disappear.

That's what's going on inside. On the outside, scars can also become inflamed, red, itchy or sensitive, just as often as they are benign. Throbbing, reduced range of motion, and a specific sensation of "creaking" at the site are also common. This can indicate infection or other more serious issues that can be addressed outside of physical therapy. Most often I see this in patients who have undergone surgery on their knees, stomach to include cesarean sections or hysterectomies, mastectomy, and discectomy.

Women have a further complication, as the scarring that they often experience is related to their pelvic health. This includes cesarean sections and episiotomies, both of which require tissue to be cut and a scar to form. Many of my female patients do not know that the pain that they continue to be in months after birth can relate directly back to those scar sites and do not realize that they need to seek treatment.

One of my biggest frustrations in my line of work is how women are not educated by their health care practitioners or doctors about the importance of scar treatment therapy. It is extremely important to treat all scars, especially when they are new. When treated promptly, the tissue underneath has a better chance of repairing, and at a quicker rate. There is less chance or risk of other issues in the future when treated, such as pelvic pain, back pain, and incontinence.

Beyond pelvic health, scarring of the breast tissue is common in women, as we previously mentioned. Scarring from breast augmentation, chemotherapy, and radiation can cause significant restrictions. This and posture affects breast tissue, leading to pain in other regions, including the chest, abdomen, shoulders, and neck.

I urge you to find an authentic Myofascial Release specialist near you to address your scars and surrounding tissue. Remember, we want to get down to the deepest layer of tissue known as the ground substance, which only authentic Barnes Myofascial Release can accomplish.

Whether it is from breast cancer, augmentation, or reduction, it is exceedingly rare for women to think of having their scars treated. It is truly saddening to hear that they never had anyone treat the scar tissue and restrictions when they step into my office with complaints of limited shoulder mobility or decreased neck motion. These women have realized that everyday life has been affected, such as blow drying their hair, brushing their teeth, or even gazing up to look at the stars in the sk, yet they do not realize why. I think about how easy the information could have been relayed, and wonder why it's not happening regularly.

All scars, no matter how small or insignificant, need treatment. The discoloring on your foot from stepping on a nail when you were eight could be the reason you struggle with urinary incontinence; the ridge line of dense tissue along your gums where you had dental surgery ten years ago could be the source of your neck pain. You are worthy of easy movement and a life unrestricted.

MEN'S HEALTH

*O*ur bodies are complex organisms made up of moving parts, organs, and a hormonal feedback system that makes it possible for us to digest, process energy, engage in respiration, and do it all over again the next day. It's a truly remarkable, organic machine when you think about it, which includes the pelvic floor components.

For men, your pelvic health is dependent upon two major players: the bowel and the bladder. As you start to age, these regions can develop problems and inconsistencies that impact your quality of life. We're going to look at some of the most popular diagnoses, including bladder control, adhesions, IBS, and interstitial cystitis, as well as solutions that are available to you.

Strong pelvic floor muscles give you control over your bladder and bowel. If your muscles are weakened these internal organs are not fully supported, causing you to have problems controlling urine, feces, and other excretions. These weakened muscles can come about from obesity, constant straining (physically intensive jobs), and constipation. These muscles stretch like a muscular trampoline from your coccyx to the pubic bone, firm and thick in composition.

In men, this muscular wall has a hole for passages to pass through, which is the urethra and anus. These muscles give us conscious control over the bladder and bowel so that we are able to release urine, feces, etc. upon command. These muscles are responsible for erectile function and ejaculation, as well as their connection to the abdominal and back muscles to support the spine. Naturally, if these muscles are weakened, you are going to have problems. We are going to look at the following conditions related to men's pelvic health that can develop from a weakening of pelvic floor muscles, as well as other happenstance scenarios.

After the age of 35, the male body starts to produce less testosterone as a result of passing the "baby making years." According to a recent study published by Harvard Medical School, testosterone is responsible for the creation and retention of muscle in men (along with other hormones), which means lower T levels can decrease the prominence of your pelvic muscles (Harvard, 2019).

Knowing that the average male testosterone rates have been decreasing at about 1.2% per year since the 1980s, as shown by researchers at New England Research Institutes, testosterone levels could very well have an impact on your pelvic health and recovery (Travison et al., 2007). So, where does this leave you? After looking at the state of your pelvis, you probably want to know if there are solutions available to you.

INTERSTITIAL CYSTITIS

*I*C, otherwise known as the bladder pain syndrome (BPS), is a chronic bladder health issue in both men and women that creates a feeling of pain in and around the bladder region. The pain can range from moderate to severe, depending upon the status of the condition. Right now, IC affects between 1 million and 4 million men, and 3 million and 8 million women in the United States (Interstitial Cystitis Association, 2019). It works like this: your bladder is a hollow, muscular organ that stores urine. When it's full, the bladder tells your brain, through nerves, that you need to pee. With IC, these signals get mixed up, causing you to "feel like" you need to pee more frequently than the average person.

Symptoms:
- Pain in your pelvis between the scrotum and anus
- Chronic pelvic pain
- A persistent need to urinate
- Pain in the bladder as it refills
- Pain during sexual intercourse

One patient of mine who suffers from interstitial cystitis has always stuck with me. He is an adult male patient who grew up in a very tense household. His dad was a professional wrestler and had a very hostile personality. There was a lot of fighting in his household, and as such, was in a constant state of tension. This patient, at a young age, began to tighten and tense his abdominal muscles anytime his father was around. First, he began to feel pain in the abdomen, and eventually, by his early 30s his bladder was affected. Because of all his bracing and tightening, he created inflammation in the bladder that started to manifest in more and more troubling symptoms. Ultimately by his mid-30s, he was living in a straight jacket of pain and uncertainty. He, at one point, was urinating up to 60 times a day. After successful MFR treatments, which he first found in California, his pain was reduced significantly and he learned how to perform self-treatment techniques for his bladder and rectum. He sought treatment at my clinic so he could better maintain the progress he achieved prior. He is now managing his symptoms, and on a pain scale of 1-10, his pain has gone to 0-2/10 on most days. He can now live a somewhat normal life. Stress can affect IC, and given his high profile career and the pressures that come along with that, he has had to learn how to soften, and not let the daily work and life stressors aggravate his symptoms. Breath work and treatment tools have been very helpful.

CHRISTOPHER'S STORY

*C*hris has been my patient for almost a year now. When I met him he was living with an 8/10 on a pain scale with abdominal pain, which he explained had been ongoing for most of his life. His experience with pain and Myofascial Release has given him exceptional insight on what it means to find relief where hope was once lost.

In my years of practice, I have noticed that it is much more difficult for my male patients to express their feelings. I'm not sure if it is mostly due to their upbringing, societal norms, or the fear of being vulnerable. I always appreciate when male patients open up because they, for the most part, keep everything locked inside, clenching their bodies and shoving down their emotions, which manifest physically as tissue restrictions and pain.

Chris shared his unique story with me, and has graciously agreed to let me share it with all of you. It is a wonderful example of how tissue holds memory and emotion, and that our bodies remember everything that ever happened to it. Read carefully, and tune into the mind-body connection that evolves within Chris.

Chris could remember feeling uneasy at home, always tightening and feeling tense at home. He shared with me that his parents would often argue with one another, his relationship with his dad being particular stressful.

His dad was a professional wrestler and was known to have a loud, and often volatile, personality. He would often yell and throw things around the home. Chris never really knew when he would be set off.

This caused him to brace and tense his stomach in anticipation of his father's reactions to various triggers.

Aside from feeling constant tension in his body at a young age, Chris didn't experience any pain until his early 30s. By then, he had built up such tightness and immense holding patterns from the constant abdominal bracing that it began to affect his bladder. He would have to urinate up to 60 times at the peak of his issues.

He sought out medical treatment and learned he had interstitial cystitis. Upon this diagnosis, Chris became a patient of mine. Over the past year, I am happy to report that he has made tremendous progress. He has reduced his symptoms from 9/10 abdominal pain, to a baseline of 3/10 on a pain scale. Most days he is actually at a 0-2/10 on a pain scale and is able to perform self-care tissue releases daily, which he is very diligent about.

By treating the emotional end of the pain, learning how to prevent and manage the emotional triggers that surface on a daily basis, as well as the physical restrictions, we have seen Chris through the worst of his symptoms and given him tools to ensure that he keeps his physical body, as well as his mind, healthy as he continues through life.

BLADDER CONTROL

*I*f you think you're suffering from a bladder control problem, consider the following signs and symptoms:

- Leaking urine during everyday activities, like bending or coughing
- Feeling a sudden urge to urinate right away
- Being unable to make it to the toilet
- Wetting yourself in your sleep

According to the National Association for Continence (NAFC), between 2% and 15% of men ages 15 to 64, and 5% to 15% of men over 60 who live at home have incontinence (Health, 2019). Therefore, it's not the most unusual of conditions, considering that as men age their muscular composition and control decreases (our muscles break down as we age and our bodies become less efficient at producing muscle-stimulant hormones, like Human Growth Hormone). Additionally, men have a prostate gland that surrounds the opening of the bladder. As men age, their prostate becomes bigger, known as prostate enlargement. It can press on your bladder, causing frequent bladder urges.

ADHESIONS

*A*dhesions are something that can happen throughout your body, known as bands of scar tissue that can cause internal organs to be stuck together when they are not supposed to be. Adhesions can come about from previous surgeries, but in this case, we are going to look at their development following a pelvic infection.

Symptoms:
- Chronic pain
- Bowel obstruction
- Inability to pass gas
- Painful bowel movements
- Emotional disorders, like depression
- Pain from moving/walking or sitting

Adhesions can only be diagnosed with some kind of diagnostic imaging or internal test, since their presence is otherwise undetected from regular doctor appointments. But, if you have adhesions obstructing your digestive system, it's safe to say, you will be blatantly aware of it.

Irritable Bowel Syndrome (IBS)

Right now in the U.S., of the 25 to 45 million people living with Irritable Bowel Syndrome (IBS), one in three is a man (Bolen, PhD, 2019). IBS causes frequent changes to bowel movements, from diarrhea one day to constipation the next, as well as abdominal swelling, bloating, and painful gas movements. The disorder has been linked to poor sleep, stress, and changes in gut bacteria that can cause digestive distress without any warnings. Additionally, IBS can be a stress-induced condition, which means considering that more people are stressed today than ever before, we are seeing this condition more prevalent.

Symptoms:
- Pain and cramping, inability to pass gas
- Diarrhea
- Constipation
- Alternating between diarrhea and constipation
- Changes in bowel movements
- Bloating
- Food intolerance
- Fatigue and difficulty sleeping

THE BRAIN-GUT
CONNECTION

Considering that many of these pelvic problems are specifically gut-related, it's also important to note that people with IBS, adhesions, etc. can also experience a heightened increase of depression and lethargic thinking. The brain-gut connection, as doctors call it, refers to the axis of your gut and mental health, with multiple studies confirming that an unwell gut can create a depressed and lethargic state of mind, as examined in a recent article published by JohnHopkins.com.

How MFR Can Help

*M*yofascial treatment in the pelvic region is not often considered by the medical community, but can significantly improve pain, posture, and range of motion in women. In men, it is even more rare. It is a mistake to diminish the importance of the pelvic region. Women's Health issues specifically are riddled with question marks and very few answers. It only makes sense that a therapy that focuses on a largely invisible organ, the fascia, is able to identify and then most importantly, treat the source of pain in women that otherwise is ignored.

When you see a therapist who specializes in MFR for a pelvic issue, you can expect a few things. First, a manual muscle assessment will be performed in order to determine whether your pain is because you lack strength, or if you require greater flexibility in the pelvic floor musculature. The therapist will also do a tissue assessment and feel for tissue that is hot, hard, or tender internally, just as they would externally. They will focus on the distinction in your deficiency because treatment will vary between them.

If you are experiencing a weakened floor as opposed to a lack of flexibility, your therapist will use your specific needs and abilities to develop a plan unique to you to get the best results while strengthening your pelvic floor. Your first line of treatment is often not Kegel exercises, despite popular belief.

For those patients who truly have a muscle power deficiency in their pelvic floor, strengthening can be the first line of defense. You will be taught how to perform these strengthening exercises properly and, surprisingly, how to perform them at the proper time. If done correctly and consistently, the cure rate is 35-80%; you will walk away with a healthy pelvic floor that is sufficiently strong where you need it.

For example, you can perform these contractions while standing in line at the grocery store, completely undetected. There should be no closing the legs together, no squeezing the bottom, and no pressing your stomach outward. All you should feel is a lifting of the pelvic floor muscles and a slight tensing or drawing in of the lower abdominal muscles. A simpler way to practice this is to try to start and stop the flow of urine. The point at which you constrict the flow is when your pelvic floor muscles are contracting. When the contraction is performed correctly, these "openings" of the body should close. No outward sign of effort should be visible with a pelvic floor muscle contraction.

While many women who have trouble controlling their pelvic floor are told to Kegel, it is important to remember that muscle tissue tightness and restriction can impact its strength. In other words, the muscle may not be working ideally because of restrictions, not because it is weak. Kegeling, therefore, can increase dysfunction by exacerbating tightness.

A person with pelvic floor weakness is often referred to Myofascial Release treatment to alleviate pelvic imbalances and restrictions, while avoiding the issues that Kegeling alone could possibly develop. After this, they may be recommended to follow up the treatment with a Kegel program.

I have had many patients complain when I recommend Kegel exercises after appropriate treatment and alignment correction has taken place. They explain that they have tried them before and they have found no difference in their pelvic health. As we discussed above, this is very likely because they have not been taught the proper method. When performed incorrectly, it is possible for incontinence to become worse, the pelvic floor to become inflamed, and pain to remain. In other words, their dysfunction is strengthened. Just like at the gym, if you exercise incorrectly while misinformed, you are not becoming stronger, you are simply endangering yourself, strengthening your dysfunction, and risking injury. Ultimately, it is best to find treatment with a physical therapist who specializes in Women's Health to guide you through a personalized regimen.

Now that we are aware of the dangers, I would encourage any female reader to attempt proper Kegel exercises right now. They are so easy that no matter where you are, you should be able to attempt them. Take a seat, if you are not already, and make sure that your legs are uncrossed. Rest your hands on your laps or at your side.

Now, begin by contracting your buttocks, thighs, and abdomen as tightly as possible. As you do this, push your feet down into the floor and clench your fists. Hold this position for ten seconds. When your ten-second hold is complete, slowly exhale and allow yourself to release the tension. You will feel your body soften.

Your next step is to only contract the gluteal muscles for ten more seconds before once again softening on an exhale. The focus will now be on your core muscles. Repeat the cycle of contracting only your abdominal core for ten seconds and softening.

Lastly, the pelvic floor. As with the rest of your body parts, contract the pelvic floor muscles by gently leaning forward in your seat and pulling in, holding the motion, squeezing the muscle for three seconds before release. Remember, it is similar to the sensation of stopping and starting the flow of urine. Repeat three more times.

Another exercise that is widely used in pelvic physical therapy, is involving vaginal weights for women. The use of weights can be helpful because it causes the vagina to contract in order to hold the weight in place and prevent it from slipping out of the body. Like any muscles, the more that it is used, the stronger it becomes.

There are other types of pelvic floor exercises, as well. These, like the weights, encourage the pelvic floor and sphincter into motion. A pelvic physical therapist can provide a program that works best for you. This program should be adhered to for best results.

The therapist may rely on biofeedback to assess your progress. Biofeedback is visual feedback that provides immediate feedback on whether or not the patient is using the correct muscles for their exercises, as well as an assessment of how much muscle activity was actually utilized and for how long. It can aide in performance of manual muscle activity.

On the other hand, your pain may be due to an overly tight or restricted pelvic floor, rather than simply a weak one. In this case, remember that Kegel exercises will only exacerbate the issue. Other treatments, such as authentic Myofascial Release, will be recommended to assist in returning normal function to that portion of your body by releasing the inflamed tissue before stabilizing and strengthening it. Your therapist can only know how to treat the pain you are experiencing by forming your treatment plan in conjunction with your unique needs.

It is important on top of all of this to remember that tissue holds memory and emotion. Essentially, your body remembers everything that ever happened to it. Holding on to things and bottling them up can, and will, create fascial lines of tension within the tissue. It can cause bladder pain and urinary frequency, as I have seen in many patients, all the way to interstitial cystitis and extreme abdominal pain. You owe it to yourself to let go of all the holding patterns and start feeling, expressing them gently. Authentic Myofascial Release can help you achieve this and so much more.

In addition to authentic Myofascial Release, taking care of your body in general will help keep your pelvic health in tip-top condition. Engage in regular exercise, eat healthy, increase range and regularity of movement, and of course, drink enough water to stay hydrated.

AGING GRACEFULLY

"The First Wealth is Health" - Ralph Waldo Emerson

When a patient realizes that they cannot pick up their grand-child, or that they can no longer work in the field that they love, they will finally decide that enough is enough and come to see someone like me, in the hope that I can help facilitate healing and give them back these experiences that they have lost. This paradigm is not exclusive to physical pain; you can also observe the concept at work emotionally.

We all have one body – and that's it. What you choose to do with your body over time will have a direct impact on how you age, how you feel, and how you look. Our bodies are resilient, no doubt, but they are not indestructible. Since we are made up of thousands of microsystems that work to keep a variety of factors in equilibrium, when we throw just one thing off, it can wreak havoc on our whole body.

As you age, this becomes more apparent. The body stops to produce tissues, collagen, and other hormones in abundance like it once did, which is why you might be worried about your health as that clock ticks forward. Additionally, all of the physical and stressful trauma you have incurred over time starts to add up. You can feel it.

It is important to note that you shouldn't wait until you can't do an activity, or are in too much pain to do what you enjoy before taking your health back into your hands. Unfortunately, I see people usually after dealing with years and years of pain or compensation. If they only listened to their body from the first warning signs, instead of ignoring or brushing it off, they would be so much better off and would not have lost as much time to their pain.

Let's look at one fitting quote by John Amaro, DC, FIACA: "You will receive one body, of which, you should never wear it out, you will have nowhere to live. You are expected to make alterations, improvements, and maintenance on a regular basis. How you feed and care for your body is paramount in how long you will operate at maximum efficiency."

He goes on to highlight that growth is merely a process of trial and error, along with experimentation. The failure to experiment, he argues, is just as detrimental as failing to invest in your body all along.

"What you make of your life is up to you. You have been given all the tools and resources you need: what you do with them is up to you. The choice is yours." We can always be learning, observing, and making changes to current habits. The decision rests entirely within ourselves and our willingness to do this. Are you willing to make a change that will help your body? Or would you rather stay committed to your current ways? In totality, it's up to you.

So, what exactly are these changes that can help you age gracefully? What even is aging gracefully in the first place?

WHAT IS AGING GRACEFULLY?

*A*ging gracefully is a euphemism we hear thrown around every day. It can mean to look old, but to embrace it. Or, it can be to show signs of aging, but still power forward with life. Essentially, aging gracefully is refusing to accept that your age defines you. Age is just a number, right?

We live in an anti-aging culture that attributes all sorts of negative connotations with getting older. In reality, it's merely a natural part of life that should be embraced with openness and understanding. The kinder you are to your body as you embark on this process, the more you will realize that your age does not define your health or vitality, whatsoever.

SELF-TREATMENT

*N*ow that we have mentioned taking care of your body to a great extent, it's time to give you some actionable techniques and information regarded to self-treatment, so you can be in the know. At its core, self-treatment is the treatment of oneself without professional supervision to alleviate an illness or condition. It's being vigilant and listening to your body when it's trying to tell you something.

If we all slow down for just a few minutes per day and close our eyes to really feel our present physical state, you'd be surprised at how obvious your body can make it when you need to address something that is off-kilter. Of course, you can't live your entire life in a doctor's office. That's why it's so important to make self-treatment part of your everyday regime. This includes both your physical and mental state. In order to preserve your mental happiness and stability, consider the following:

1. Eat healthy brain foods: Researchers have proven, time and time again, that junk food raises our depression risk. If you eat this kind of garbage your entire life, it will become part of the fabric of your body. Treat your brain to delicious, nutritious, and brain-stimulating foods, like berries or avocados, when you can.
2. Talk to people: Isolation was never the intention for humans. Be sure to make time for some chat and bonding with people every single day, whether it's family, coworkers, or friends.

3. Do something you love each day: Aging doesn't have to be miserable. Pick one thing you love, like painting, and make time for it every day. Feed your joy and happiness.

Of course, there are a million other things you can do to preserve your mental platform as you age gracefully. But what about your physical body?

1. Get enough sleep: Sleep is arguably the most important thing we do for our bodies every single day. From your brain to your muscle performance, our bodies need restful sleep. That's probably why people who sleep less than 6-hours per night are more likely to die early than their rested counterparts, according to researchers at the University of Warwick and Federico II University Medical School in Naples, who analyzed 16 studies involving a total of 1.3 million people before reaching their conclusions.
2. Reduce stress: Although stress might seem mental, it can bring about a slew of bodily conditions, like arthritis, inflammation, chronic pain, and the list goes on. As you age, if you continue to shoulder immense stress every single day, it will start to wear away at your body.
3. Exercise: We were not meant to be sedentary creatures. Our bodies were designed to walk, run, jump, squat, and everything in-between. The more you exercise as you age, the more agile your body, muscles, and joints will feel.

This last point of exercise is more important than you might realize. Why? Because it's related to Myofascial Release, which is a secret aging treatment you're going to want to know more about. We feel it's our duty to make sure you understand your body and what's available at your disposal as you age with time (Dartmouth-hitchcock.org, 2019).

THE SECRET TO AGING

"Years may wrinkle the skin, but to give up enthusiasm wrinkles the soul" - Samuel Ullman

John F. Barnes, PT, has brought to light the many ways that Myofascial Release can help ease the strains of aging by targeting the fascia. His methods have helped me help my patients in their golden years continue the activities that bring them joy.

Myofascial Release and myofascial freedom involves a multidimensional approach and technique. The ultimate goal is to lengthen the shortened fascial tissue that can bunch up as you age. This includes accumulated trauma, physical and emotional, repetitive motions that may develop because of habitual actions, and failure to exercise, an unfortunate side effect of getting older for many people.

As Myofascial Release is performed on the body, it unwinds neuromuscular holding patterns while facilitating structural alignment. In layman's terms, it stretches out your fascia so you can enjoy a limber quality of life again. Of course, simply stretching your body isn't going to fix this problem. Stretching is great for keeping your muscles elongated, etc., but it won't cure the trauma inflicted to your connective tissue. Traditional stretching wraps and pulls tissue around joint fulcrums. That's where Myofascial Release comes into the picture.

Myofascial Release stretches the structures three-dimensionally, telescoping the myofascial tissues and subsequent bony spaces. This is what separates it from traditional stretching–the application of counter pressures and fulcrums on tissues.

Myofascial Release is considered to be the highest order of therapeutic artistry today. In addition to being effective in the resolution of pain and headaches, while also restoring movement, it's also an effective tool that enables a person to enhance their awareness potential. In this case, it helps a person fight off the signs and feeling of aging. Regardless of your personal, physical, or mental trauma, as well as your body's current state, everyone could stand to benefit from Myofascial Release.

ANNE'S STORY

"*A*ging gracefully was something I made a conscious decision to do. I was turning 50 and it was time to take stock. After years of child rearing, completing college degrees, operating a state certified family home daycare business, plus all that family life entails, I came to the realization that I needed to make my health a priority.

My youngest child was in high school and I had taken a teaching position in Providence, RI so I had more time for myself, as the day care business was a 12-hour a day job. The starting point was to lose the extra pounds that had crept on over the years. I started to watch what I was eating and took advantage of my YMCA membership. The results of my efforts were gradual, but consistent. As the weeks went by the pounds came off and I was feeling stronger. The best part was that I had so much more energy!

As a 50th birthday gift, I received a membership to the Appalachian Mountain Club (AMC), something I had wanted since I was in high school. I grew up in the White Mountains of New Hampshire where hiking, skiing, ice skating, and biking were activities I participated in on a regular basis. It was time for me to get back to the things I loved doing as a child. With my regained health I found that I was once again on the slopes of Loon Mountain, climbing 4000-foot mountains as well as smaller ones, hiking from hut to hut on Franconia Ridge and the Presidential Range, and doing local RI hikes. There was also a 14-day AMC adventure to hike in the Olympic and Cascade Mountain Ranges of Washington. Instead of biking, I took up kayaking. With the help of AMC volunteers, I learned to paddle a 17-foot fiberglass Wilderness System sea kayak. It wasn't long before I was an AMC kayak leader myself. I've paddled all over Narragansett Bay in RI, the Kittery in ME, Bar Harbor and Knuble Bay areas and the Saco River, the Stonington, CT area, as well as Morro Bay and Santa Cruz Island in CA. I was at 'the top of my game,' so to speak.

In the fall of 2006, I had surgery for carpal tunnel on my right hand, and several vein surgeries on both legs, but mainly the right leg. That is when things started to go wrong. Over the years, I have had several surgical procedures with no problems. However, this time something was not right. I started having more and more pain in my joints and felt my energy waning. My neck and shoulders were tight, and I was losing range of motion in many areas of my body. I saw a chiropractor and had regular deep tissue massages, until I could not handle the pain. My doctor was saying it was arthritis, while checking for MS and Lupus. I didn't feel like it was any of these. One day in May of 2007, fed up with the pain and lack of mobility, I went to a walk-in clinic in my town. There, I finally got a diagnosis that made sense. It was Lyme disease, most likely contracted in the fall of 2006. That was almost six months without proper diagnosis and treatment. I was put on what would be a two-year regiment of various antibiotics, some being very potent. There were supplements and mega probiotics to balance out the antibiotics. I continued many of my activities, but with much pain and discomfort. It got worse before it got better. After two years of treatment I discontinued antibiotics and was moving and feeling much better, on my way back to 'normal.' That was in June of 2009.

Almost a month to the day of discontinuing treatment for Lyme, I received another tick bite. While having lunch on the top of Indian Head in Lincoln, NH a friend noticed a large, red circle on the back of my left leg. The previous few days I had had a headache and was feeling achy, but didn't make the connection. When I got back to RI, I went directly to the clinic that had first diagnosed me. The doctor confirmed that it was Lyme and pointed out the satellite blotches on other parts of my body.

Once again, I was on an antibiotic regimen. This time the joints hurt even more than before. The pain was worse in my feet, and moved all the way up through my legs to my back, neck, and shoulders. I continued my activities, though it was difficult and painful. I thank my friends for providing encouragement and helping me out in any way they could. On hikes, I was the slowest one and often needed help getting in and out of my kayak. If I had given up and just stayed home, I'm sure depression would have set in and I would have another problem to deal with. One thing I knew was that I should keep moving.

After my second two years on antibiotics I felt something was wrong. I was developing neuropathy in both legs from my knees to my toes. This was a side effect of the antibiotic I was on. I discontinued taking it and waited to see what would happen. My primary care doctor said if the neuropathy was going to reverse at all it would take up to six months. It took almost a year and there is still some in my left toes. Balance was difficult and I was doing less and less of my outdoor activities. Teaching a full day pre-k class of up to 30 children was taking all my energy. I took a hard fall on my tailbone at work, had surgery for a hammer toe, as well as snapped the T-band in my right leg, which happened while at a Wilderness First Aid Training class, just added to my physical problems. Everything hurt from head to toe. I had surgery on my right knee for a torn meniscus and was told I would most likely need a knee replacement. I had had physical therapy for bursitis in my hip and for the knee surgery. It wasn't enough. I felt I needed therapy on my entire body, but my insurance would not cover any more than the minimal therapy on diagnosed problem areas. I didn't know where to turn, but I wasn't giving in.

It was at this same time that my sister was going to physical therapy for knee pain. From her first visit she had positive results. With each visit the pain subsided until she was pain-free. The interesting thing was that the therapist said he was using Myofascial Release therapy on her. I had never heard of that type of therapy, so I did a little research. It sounded like just what I needed. However, it was not easy to find a therapist that was practicing Myofascial Release Therapy here in RI. Even if I did find one, my insurance was not going to pay because there was no specific diagnosis, I was able to do self-care, was mobile, and able to go to work. Head to toe pain that was negatively affecting my entire life was not enough to qualify for insurance coverage.

With much excitement and hope I discovered the website of Dr. Jessica Papa. She is a well-trained Myofascial Release practitioner and was taking new clients. Insurance or no insurance, I was going to give this a try. At that time, Jessica's practice was a traveling one. She came right to my home for treatment. From the very first meeting we had a connection. She did a thorough evaluation to assess exactly what condition my body was in. Aside from the pain in my entire body, I had very limited range of motion in my right knee, hips, arms, and neck. When asked to raise my arms I could only get my elbows as high as my shoulders. My neck would only turn a few inches in either direction. My right knee only had about half its range of motion. There was a great deal of inflammation in my body. When she asked me to lift my leg off the table while on my back, I could not do it. After hearing my medical history, she told me that my problems most likely were the result of years of dealing with Lyme disease. This is the same conclusion that I had come to on my own, but had no idea how to move forward.

On April 26, 2016, I began an incredible journey to good health with Dr. Jessica Papa as my guiding light. Having experienced my share of physical therapy in the past, I knew that there could be discomfort involved and that I would have homework to do. With every visit (they were weekly for some time) I felt my body reacting in positive ways. The exercises she gave me to do on my own were challenging and as I mastered each set there were always new ones waiting to be learned. It wasn't long before I was feeling less pain, gaining more mobility, and was able to be more active. Every week I looked forward to our time together and what a relief it would bring.

Here I am in 2019, at the age of 70, pain-free and active. I'm doing the things I enjoy, like taking an eight mile hike in Letchworth State Park, NY to view the three magnificent waterfalls there. I still see Jessica once a month for a wellness checkup. I feel the checkup is important because I do not want to lose what I have gained. To stay on track, I wear a Fit Bit and walk at least four miles a day, climb ten flights of stairs, and am active for 40 minutes a day. To that, I add an hour or so of exercises I am assigned to do at home, which I now do every other day. I follow a Med-DASH diet for the most part and practice yoga daily, as well as attend a class once a week, when possible. Not a day goes by that I am not thankful for having met Jessica and experienced the power of Myofascial Release Therapy. The lady has magical powers! I wish everyone in pain would discover Myofascial Release Therapy. The world would be a better, healthier place and far fewer drugs, as well as surgeries, would be needed."

MYSTERY ILLNESS: FIBROMYALGIA

*F*ibromyalgia has landed itself at the top of the mystery illness list, being a chronic pain condition that doctors simply cannot pinpoint a "cure" for. According to the National Fibromyalgia Association, it leaves about 10 million Americans in pain, at a loss for words every year, attacking different tissues and nerves. It results in severe pain, or worse, temporarily immobility (Silver et al., 2016).

At its base, fibromyalgia causes widespread pain, fatigue, and other types of discomfort. Many symptoms resemble those of arthritis, although fibromyalgia attacks soft tissue, and not just the joints. Common symptoms include: widespread pain, jaw pain and stiffness, headaches, irregular sleeping patterns, restless leg syndrome, painful menstrual periods, irritable bowel syndrome, sensitivity to cold or heat, fatigue, and difficulties with concentration.

There is much discussion in the medical community. We ask: is fibromyalgia related to chronic fatigue syndrome? Is it simply chronic pain and headaches related to pelvic or menstrual pain and PMS? Is it a trigger of these other conditions? A symptom? Are they related?

In reality, these are all simply different labels we have placed on a common denominator, known as unrecognized myofascial restrictions. These restrictions do not show up in all of the standard tests that are now performed, nor have most health professionals been made aware of the process of recognizing them.

This leaves millions of people in pain and with questions, wondering if they will ever be able to find a solution that is right for them. Fibromyalgia is not something with a black-and-white answer. It's incredibly frustrating, defeating, and of course, painful for those living with it.

That's why we're here to propose a solution to this kind of condition. We don't accept simply living with it for the rest of your life and hoping it will get better. We're going to look at different kinds of triggers for fibromyalgia that you might not even realize are related, as well as a tangible solution that can protect your body.

TRAUMA

oth physical and mental trauma can trigger fibromyalgia. There have been multiple studies that have confirmed physical trauma, like childbirth or a car accident, can bring on fibromyalgia and reoccurring, chronic pain (Adler, 2019).

Chronic stress and mental pressures can also bring about chronic pain conditions, like fibromyalgia, confirming that the disease can be derived entirely from the health and state of our minds (Gupta and Silman, 2004). This may be a contributing factor in why many veterans diagnosed with post-traumatic stress disorder meet the criteria of fibromyalgia. In fact, in a study conducted by the American College of Rheumatology in 1990, it was found that 49% of veterans met the criteria, confirming that mental stress can be a huge trigger in the disease.

Childhood trauma can bring around fibromyalgia, as well. A Tel Aviv University study on the effects of trauma in an individual's earlier years, finds that fibromyalgia syndrome may be a consequence of post-traumatic physical and psychological distress associated with childhood abuse–especially sexual abuse. As the study states, "We now know that severe emotional stress, such as that caused by sexual abuse, can induce chronic brain injury. These non-healing brain wounds may explain certain unremitting long-term physical and psychological disorders, like fibromyalgia" (Shira, 2012).

AUTONOMIC NERVOUS SYSTEM

*A*nother common cause of fibromyalgia is an over-activation of the autonomic nervous system. Otherwise known as your sympathetic nervous system, this system is your fight-or-flight response to things in your world. On the other hand, your parasympathetic nervous system is what relaxes you and tells your body to calm down.

When you're on your feet all day, working hard, or stressing out, your sympathetic nervous system starts to flare. But, when you sit down to digest a meal, the parasympathetic system kicks in to lower the fight-or-flight response levels in your body. If you get ready for an afternoon meeting and start to feel a little nervous, this sympathetic nervous system goes back up. And the cycle continues.

For people with fibromyalgia, this sympathetic nervous system is always at a heightened state. This is where it can relate to trauma. Major stressful events, or a series of events, can rev up the system so high, that when the parasympathetic system kicks back in, it's unable to counteract the first system and bring it back down.

Most people are aware of the phenomenon that is commonly referred to as the fight-or-flight response, the reaction that most individuals have when confronted with trauma or danger. This includes even those who do not suffer from illnesses, such as fibromyalgia. It is largely a product of your autonomic nervous system.

People and animals, when confronted with danger, will immediately react. When you're stuck in fight-or-flight mode, your senses are much more heightened. Your pupils dilate, the hair on your arms stands on end to enhance your sense of contact, and your heart rate speeds up. Instead of needing to activate, say five muscles, to get a movement done, your body is now using 20 and a few extra joints. That is why those with fibromyalgia jump back at the sense of touch. Their nerves are so heightened that it can be processed as pain, whereas in a parasympathetic state, this would never happen.

Their reaction will often be a variation of these two responses: become aggressive in the hope that the source of danger can defeated, or flee. These responses are controlled by the autonomic nervous system and occur whether the person or animal is aware. There is one other option that is rarely spoken about, and that is the freeze response.

In the case of an animal who has been put into a threatening position, the duration of immobility brought on by the body's freeze response is normally time-limited. The animal then naturally emerges from it when the threat has either been eliminated or they have been removed from the situation. When they do, an enormous amount of energy is discharged in the form of shaking, profuse sweating, and deep breathing. As the energy is dissipated, they return to their typical state of calm alertness.

In this, humans are different. When a human is triggered into a freeze response, the body does not easily and naturally resolve the reaction. The supercharged energy that is released from within an animal does the exact opposite in humans. The human body, instead, locks that energy within the nervous system and imprisons the emotion and trauma. This results in a vicious cycle of fear and immobility that takes over, preventing the response from completing naturally. When not allowed to resolve, these responses form the symptoms of trauma and present themselves in a pain response.

Myofascial Release allows for a completion of this instinctive cycle in a safe, natural, and effective manner. Working in reverse, Myofascial Release and Myofascial Unwinding start with present day restrictions and compensations.

YOUR MIND AND HOLDING PATTERNS

*A*s you can see, fibromyalgia sounds pretty exhausting. Your body feels like it is constantly being attacked, which can send you into a mental exhaustion of constantly feeling on "edge" and needing to defend yourself.

Your brain exists in two levels, keeping your body in preparation for what it needs to know. There is a conscious level, of which you tell your body what to do: pick up a fork, go to the bathroom, etc. But, there is an unconscious level as well. This unconscious level is what is stimulated negatively by fibromyalgia.

If your brain becomes wired to be "scared of something," or anticipatory that someone is always going to hurt you, this unconscious level will always be on the defensive. In order to minimize energy expenditure, your brain will go into what's known as a holding pattern, which is something very common in nature. While in this pattern, it naturally starts to perpetuate the fight-or-flight response without elevating it to any level of consciousness. This then makes it harder to break out of the fibromyalgia cycle.

Additionally, there's also a physical component to note here. Your brain can swell if you chronically suffer from fibromyalgia. Several studies have found the presence of neuroinflammation in the brains of patients with fibromyalgia, due to an overdrive of nerve activity

(Bäckryd, 2017). This is the reasoning behind why so many will complain of chronic headaches and migraines.

As you can see, it is all interrelated. Whether it was physical trauma that started your mental holding pattern or the permanent fight-or-flight mode that resulted from mental distress, once fibromyalgia kicks in, it can be hard to break.

MYOFASCIAL RELEASE

*A*t this time, we know that the best thing for fibromyalgia is movement and exercise. Specifically, submaximal exercise and effort–doing some movement and engagement without wiping your body out. This is where Myofascial Release comes into the picture. It can provide significant relief of pain and headaches, as well as the restoration of motion.

Fascia surrounds and infuses every organ, duct, nerve, blood vessel, bone, and muscle in the pelvic cavity. As we have seen, fascia tightens after trauma, inflammatory processes, poor posture, and childbirth–with the ability to exert over 2,000 pounds per square inch of strength on pain-sensitive structures.

"The primary communication system in our body is fascia," says Barnes, "People have been calling fascia an insulator for years, when in reality, it's more like fiber optics. When trauma or dysfunction befalls a person, fascial sheaths in the body end up glued together, becoming unyielding. This is where the pain begins. Myofascial Release is another dimension to massage and bodywork that helps to create a more long-lasting result."

Although massage has been proven to help in some capacity, it only relieves about 20% of the fascial system, otherwise known as the elastic and muscular components of the myofascial complex. To reach the other 80%, Myofascial Release has to be pursued, which is why Myofascial Release has proven to help tremendously with this type of disease.

This kind of practice is about feeling the depths of a person's body and how it responds to the pressure of Myofascial Release. As fascia releases, it almost feels like taffy stretching. It's not about forcing tissue or digging deep. It's about approaching the tissue with patience to avoid triggering any fight-or-flight response that will flare the fibromyalgia pain again.

If you are suffering from fibromyalgia, I urge you to consider adding Myofascial Release to your regular treatment. There is no other method that will help soften and unwind fascia and no other method that will bring the same, long lasting relief. It is time to find the root of your chronic pain.

THERESA'S STORY

Theresa is a patient of mine and has been for five years. She was a stranger to me when I first met her years ago in a clinic I worked at before opening Arancia. When I first began at this clinic, it was policy to shadow the clinic owner in order to see how he treated patients.

Theresa had been one of the patients I would observe him treating. I will never forget when it went silent in the room during one of her sessions, just for a brief moment. The silence seemed to be too intense for him to handle and he had to break it by talking about another random, unimportant topic.

In my mind, I was thinking how similar this experience felt to my last place of work. Each owner had been so disconnected and off-center. When you are truly centered, you can be silent and focus fully on the patient, feeling through your hands and letting your patient get the absolute, most benefit from their time with you.

So, as I mentioned, Theresa was not my patient originally, but one day she appeared on my schedule. I so badly wanted to take over as her primary therapist because I knew she needed myofascial treatment. This was my chance!

Like many patients that I would occasionally treat at this former clinic, Theresa showed up in my treatment room, ready to chat about day to day occurrences, and had questions about me and my personal life. She generally wanted to keep talking since up until then, that's what her therapy sessions consisted of, talking and "getting fixed."

She was full of questions for me as I began to explain the fascial system. I could tell she was in deep thought, much like I had been at my first Myofascial Release class. I could see a glimmer of hope in her, as she was starting to let her guard down, and letting me begin *my way* of treatment on her skin! She was so used to her former therapist working over her clothes, manipulating her body, and yapping away.

When I began, I could hear the excitement in her voice, exclaiming to me that no one has ever touched her pain in this way before, that it felt so right, that I was actually connected to what she was feeling. We were off to a good start, but it would take several sessions before I could fully explain this amazing system (fascia) in our bodies.

She is a stubborn woman, and that is something that I have always loved about her, probably because she reminds me of my own grandmother. She does things her way, just like my Gram did. Oh, and she always greets me with a big hug when she comes in for her appointment! She has had a unique experience with battling fibromyalgia and has found relief in Myofascial Release. She was kind enough to recount her experience for us. This is her story.

From Theresa

"Fibromyalgia! What is that? Years ago, I couldn't even say the word, let alone figure out what it meant or how to deal with it. Like any mother of three boys, my life was very active (before fibromyalgia). I remember trips to the beach, long bike rides, hikes, camping, making huge snowmen, baseball, basketball, swimming (or trying to; I sink like a rock), and mountain climbing in the White Mountains, even climbing Mt. Washington! I was always cooking and baking. My cookie jar became famous among my sons and their friends. It was always full of delicious chocolate chip cookies. I worked in human resources as a personnel assistant and somehow found time to go back to school to work on finishing up my bachelor's degree. I always loved riding my bike. I live near the East Bay Bike Path, and every chance I got, I was out exploring on my bike.

For the first few years after my hysterectomy, I had no idea who I was or what I had become. I didn't know its name yet, but it took over my life. I had no energy. My bike sat in the basement collecting dust; my cookie jar was empty. I left school because I started having panic attacks. My whole body hurt. I was completely physically and emotionally drained. Doctor after doctor told me that there was nothing wrong with me and that I should probably 'give counseling a try.' Finally, when I was 50, my primary care doctor referred me to a rheumatologist who diagnosed me with fibromyalgia. That was 23 years ago.

My two oldest boys were 27 and 25, my youngest son was just 13 years old. Everyone was living at home with my husband and I, and they all were suffering with me. My rheumatologist told me to get back to aerobic exercise, and put me on some medication. I didn't last very long on the medication, as it gave me nightmares. And as far as aerobic exercise goes, I was thrilled since my bike would soon stop collecting dust. Even then, things had to change.

I liked riding my bike fast. It was a thrill for me to pass other bikers on the bike path and leave them in the dust. But I could no longer ride like that. I had to pace myself. My motto had to be, 'listen to my body and stop when it tells you it is time to stop.' I just wasn't ready for that. I wanted my old life back. Maybe I needed a second opinion.

Disappointment after disappointment (with traditional treatment) left me with no choice but to try alternative medicine. Over the years, I've tried many different medications, three different holistic doctors, Reiki, four different massage therapists, at least ten different physical therapists, cranial sacral therapy, water aerobics, yoga, pain management doctors, chiropractors, acupuncture, and orthopedic doctors. Some things I gave up right away, others I stuck with for quite a while, but all had the same results—minor relief, major flare-ups.

I stumbled upon Dr. Jess, I'm convinced, by the grace of God. I had been seeing a physical therapist for my hip and back when I was assigned to her one day when my regular therapist was not available. After just one treatment, I asked to be moved to Dr. Jess's schedule. That's how I was introduced to Myofascial Release Therapy.

At first I was skeptical, but soon became impressed with my new therapist (and therapy). I had so many questions and Dr. Jess was so patient. She answered every one of my questions explicitly and to my understanding. I learned how to breathe and relax to get the most out of my treatments. I learned how to use the ball to release the deep layers of fascia that caused me so much pain. I learned that I needed to slow down and realize my limitations. Most importantly, I learned that I needed to change my negative thoughts into positive ones.

Without Myofascial Release Therapy, I am convinced I would be hunched over and in a wheelchair. MFR gave me back the ability to walk in the woods, cook for my beloved family, travel with my husband, and enjoy my incredible grandchildren. It gave me back my life, not in the same way it was, but in a different way, a way that is so much better for someone who finally learned how to pronounce and spell the word 'fibromyalgia.'"

Why Your TMJ Pain May Be Indicative of a Greater Body Alignment Problem

*I*s your jaw sore? Do you experience difficulty when opening your mouth? Do you experience regular, mild headaches? Does your jaw click or make any other noises when chewing tough foods? Do you experience pain or stiffness in your jaw upon awakening? Therapy of the craniosacral mechanism, which contains the temporomandibular (jaw) joint, is very important.

Having distortion or restrictions of cranial motion can cause illnesses until the physiological balance is restored. A person with craniomandibular dysfunction may experience unusual head and neck symptoms. This discomfort can be a result of head and neck trauma. Each accident in a patient's life can have a distorting and restricting effect on the cranial mechanism. Accidents create tension in the cranial dural membranes and disrupt the cranial bone motion. This tighter mechanism causes pressure on the brain, spinal cord, and nerves resulting in many symptoms and a more restricted craniosacral mechanism. When you think of headaches, jaw pain, migraines, and other kinds of inflammations that can afflict an otherwise healthy individual, it is easy to assume that it may be related to something like lack of hydration, or some sort of physical trauma, like a collision. While these symptoms may be partly attributed to such incidents, there is an unseen, just as likely culprit right under your nose.

The temporomandibular (TMJ) joint is the natural mechanism of your skeletal system that connects your jawbone to your skull. It works as a hinge, coming off of each side of your jaw, allowing freedom of movement at that specific place of your face. It is vastly important to everyday tasks like talking, drinking, and eating. What I want to talk about is what happens when this amazing little piece of the anatomy becomes unaligned or damaged.

Anyone with a TMJ disorder will almost always experience pain in the jaw, as well as the muscles surrounding it that control jaw movement. Some other signs that you may be suffering from a misalignment or other issue with your TMJ are:

- Pain or tenderness of your jaw
- Pain in one or both of the TMJs
- Aching pain in and around the ear; might feel like a perpetual earache
- Aching facial pain
- Locking of the TMJ
- Difficulty opening and closing mouth
- Grinding of teeth while sleeping
- The disorder can also cause an audible clicking sound each time you open your mouth widely.

Some common conditions that can respond to treatment of the cranial system include:

- Headaches
- Neck pain
- "Fibro Fog"
- Decreased concentration and memory
- Depression and Anxiety

- Neurological symptoms, such as tone, tremors, numbness, and tingling

It can be hard to determine the cause of TMJ pain. You can have origins from anything, from genetics and arthritis to a specific jaw injury. TMJ can also be brought about by people who tend to clench their jaw and grind their teeth, otherwise known as bruxism. Typically, TMJ disorders can occur if the disk erodes or moves out of alignment, if the cartilage becomes damaged by arthritis, or other larger alignment problems (stemming from your pelvis).

The good news is that TMJ can be somewhat managed without intervention. If you suspect you are grinding your teeth or clenching your jaw, don't rush to get a night guard fitted by your dentist. I would, instead, encourage you first to see an authentic Myofascial Release therapist near you. An advanced therapist can address long-standing holding patterns and restrictions that are affecting the alignment and function of your jaw, which are causing the grinding. You may even be surprised to find that the imbalance started in your pelvis, where your body gets its center of gravity from. If you aren't level there, everything above has to compensate and do a job that it wasn't built to do in the first place. Over time, it causes microtraumas to the entire body.

There is a simple reason for this. Using a mouthguard or other hardware will help with the pain and prevent further damage by eliminating the grinding of your teeth. It will not, however, treat the reason you are grinding them in the first place. It may even cause new symptoms that weren't there before. If you only treat the symptoms, you will effectively be saddling yourself with a sleep aid and risking damage elsewhere that may not be so easily reversed.

BILATERAL CONFIGURATION

*D*id you know that the jaw is the only bilateral joint in the human body? This means that the temporomandibular joint (TMJ) moves together, both sides as one. Again, this is important in context of the body as a whole because when the pelvis is not level, it can contribute to asymmetries all the way up to the jaw and cranial bones. Your jaw can be a reflection of a much larger imbalance in your greater skeletal frame, which is why relief for TMJ and other injuries that affect alignment can be experienced through the careful release and preservation of the connective (fascial) tissue.

Myofascial Release treatment for the Craniosacral Mechanism and TMJ structure includes gentle manipulation of the cranial tissues to release the tension in the mechanism. Specific palpation of the bones, acting as levers, will also release tension. This will direct the cranial tissues into a position of greater ease and less stress. Afterwards, individual bones will feel more symmetrical and mobile.

A very common cause of this, and subsequent domino effect issues, is car accidents.

According to the Association for Safe International Road Travel, it is estimated that nearly 1.25 million people are killed in road crashes within the U.S. every single year, which means that about 3,287 people die per day. Of those that are not killed, an additional 20-50 million are injured or disabled. Ranked as the 9th leading cause of death in the U.S., the numbers are getting worse with the arrival of texting.

You can expect to experience the following after an auto collision:

- Whiplash
- Spinal misalignment
- Paralysis
- Numbness
- Back pain
- PTSD
- Neck/shoulder pain or stiffness
- Headaches

DONNA'S STORY–FROM CANCER TO VICTOR

*C*ancer is something that affects people, families, and patients around the world as we struggle to find a cure and help those that are fighting for their lives. With over 100 million people as of 2017 struggling with this frustrating disease, if this is you, know that you are not alone.

In this testimonial, we're going to look at the story of Donna, a cancer survivor struggling with TMJ as a result of her radiation and cancer treatments. Living with chronic pain that makes it hard for her to talk at times, Donna is enduring burning, stabbing, shooting sensations, and sharp pains that are worsened at times with no warning.

Additionally, eating thick, dense food has become nearly impossible, as Donna can only open her mouth 3-4mm instead of the typical 40mm. Swallowing is also painful, due to the increased dryness in her throat and subsequent loss of taste and appetite. These limitations force her to cut down on the amount of work she is able to do at times, as well as makes it hard for her to communicate with people in a personal and business setting.

Donna has learned how to tune into her tissue restrictions, becoming even more aware and in-tune with what is going on in her body, and stays present during her sessions so that her body can receive the healing that it needs. A wonderful quality that Donna possesses is the ability to see the positive in everything. Despite having had to deal with cancer, the ramifications of treatment, and living in constant pain, she has chosen to be thankful and grateful for the life that she lives. Her personality could light up any room; she is a joy to be around. Donna has become part of the Arancia family, and truly embodies all that is Myofascial Release, as she has experienced first-hand relief in her own body and mind. I am lucky to know her.

From Donna

"I was diagnosed with cancer of the mouth and neck, receiving a serious prognosis in regards to my future. I knew I needed to work with a professional to give my body the fighting chance it deserves, which is when I started to consider physical therapy services.

No one prepares you for receiving the news that you have cancer. And no one especially prepares you for losing function of your jaw–something that is actually much more central to our daily lives and comfort than we might realize. For awhile, I didn't know what to do. I didn't know if I was going to make it.

After undergoing six months of radiation in my jaw and neck, it left me with the inability to open my mouth wide enough to eat or talk without severe pain. As you can imagine, it impacted my everyday life, my ability to connect and talk with people, my ability to socialize, my ability to sleep soundly, and my ability to work. I knew I needed to be proactive about it.

At the time, my oral surgeon in Boston recommended that I select a Myofascial Release specialist. He knew one in Rhode Island, and put me in contact with Dr. Jess. I am so grateful that he did this, because upon meeting with Dr. Jess, I started to feel hope and encouragement for my future–like there was a possibility that I could be comfortable living life as a cancer survivor. I finally thought to myself–I could feel like a normal, living, breathing human being again.

I started the healing process in November 2016. Since then, there has been significant changes in my ability to eat and talk with less pain. What used to be excruciating is, at times, manageable, and at other times, pain-free. The more I worked with this clinic, the more I realized that miracles are possible. I couldn't stop telling everyone I knew about my healing journey.

The clinic works with me as an individual and my personal requirements, treating me like the only patient in the world. Dr. Jess has been brilliant when practicing techniques suitable for my specific medical requirements. I could cry when I think any further about what this team has done for me.

I want anyone to know, especially any cancer survivor, that this clinic is one that will work with you. You won't be just another number shoved in and out of the waiting room. They are ready to treat you as the whole package. I don't know where I'd be without them."

CAR ACCIDENTS

Car accidents are one of the top five ways your fascia can become dehydrated. Remember that fascia is largely water based. When it goes through a forceful motion, like a car accident, the fascia provides your body with a great deal of shock absorption to protect you. It is why we don't automatically break bones or tear muscles in a crash. Instead, our fascial tissue gets dried out and we feel pain in more than one place. Usually, the whole body feels stiff and tight. This is why it is key to have your whole body treated, not just pieces and parts.

WHIPLASH

The most basic definition of whiplash is that it is simply a neck injury due to a forceful, rapid, back-and-forth movement of the neck, which is what earned it the "whip" name (like cracking a whip). Whiplash is most common following rear-end auto accidents, but it can also be brought about by sports accidents, physical abuse, or physical trauma. Whiplash can happen to any person, of any age, body type, or size.

Common signs of whiplash include:

- Neck pain
- Neck sprain/strain
- Stiffness
- Headaches
- Loss of range of motion in the neck
- Tenderness in the shoulder, upper back, or arms
- Tingling or numbness in the arms
- Fatigue
- Dizziness

Most people suffering from whiplash get better a few weeks after the point of trauma. However, that's not the case for everyone. Many people can have chronic neck pain and other long-lasting complications that can impact their lives forever. It's important to see a doctor if you have been involved in some kind of whiplash incident, as anything related to head or neck damage can be potentially dangerous.

It's also very important to keep in mind that although the neck goes through a coup-contra-coup type of motion in a car accident, that is not the only thing that can be affected. All parts of your body can feel the aftereffects of the trauma long after your have healed on the surface.

CERVICOGENIC HEADACHES

*H*eadaches are one of the most common physical complaints I hear from patients and can be one of the more frustrating to manage. Headaches refer to pain in any part of the head, but there are many types. Some types of headaches include tension type or migraines. Headache pain can be caused by a migraine disorder, neck trauma, head injury, jaw disorders, neck dysfunction, or tension pain. There are numerous pain-sensitive structures that exist in the cervical (upper neck) and occipital (back of head) regions. The point where your skull and cervical vertebra meet includes regions that are pain-generating, including the lining of the cervical spine, joints, ligaments, cervical nerve roots, and vertebral arteries that pass through the cervical vertebral bodies.

Cervicogenic headaches originate here. They are caused by distortion or compression of these associated components of the body. These types of headaches differ from ones that manifest from simple neck pain, in that there is evidence of a disorder or lesion within the cervical spine or soft tissue of the neck.

People that suffer from cervicogenic headaches typically experience:

- Reduced range of motion in the neck
- Worsening of headaches with certain movements of the neck
- One sided headaches

- Pain radiating from the neck/back of the head up to the front, behind the eyes

It is common for cervicogenic headaches to mimic the symptoms of migraines, which can include:

- Feeling sick to your stomach
- Throwing up
- Sensitivity to bright light
- Sensitivity to loud sounds
- Blurry vision

While some headaches are harmless and resolve on their own, frequently recurring headaches can affect your ability to complete daily tasks and impact your quality of life.

TREATMENT

*M*yofascial restrictions can produce enormous pressure on pain-sensitive structures like we described above. Therefore, a malfunction of the fascial system can create a binding down of the fascia, which exerts pressure on nerves, muscles, bones, and organs. This also means that through the targeting of this fascia, relief is possible for many people in pain today.

Myofascial Release treatment will include careful compression combined with stretch for a minimum of five minutes so the body may return to homeostasis. Therefore, MFR techniques are utilized for a wide-range of diagnoses including pain, movement, restriction, spasm, neurological dysfunction, head injury, pelvic pain, headaches, TMJ, sports injuries, chronic fatigue, and the list goes on. Through something as simple as improving your movement, flexibility, and agility your chronic pain manifestations can be a thing of the past.

Working together with your therapist, a plan of care can be designed to meet your goals and work to correct the problems directly causing your pain. This will include improving your neck mobility and posture. Simple lifestyle changes in your work space can also help prevent headaches. This includes:

1. Using a headset or speaker, instead of holding a regular phone.
2. Adjusting your computer screen so that it is no lower than the level of your eyes.

3. Finding an appropriate desk chair that keeps you up straight and supported.

Excessive sitting at work can also lead to headaches, neck, and/or back pain. Sitting most of the day leads to strained posture and tension in the neck and lower back, leading to tension headaches. Another trigger is staring at a computer screen all day. The strain on your eyes and the blue light causes headaches. It's important to limit your time staring at a computer as much as possible and take frequent breaks.

CRANIAL SACRAL THERAPY

Related to Myofascial Release, cranial sacral techniques will also be of assistance in these instances. This method requires specialists to work with the bones of the skull and the pelvis, protecting the spinal cord between the two. This therapy involves applying gentle pressure and manipulation to the joints in the skull, spine, and pelvis, which improves the circulation of cerebrospinal fluid to help the body heal and realign itself. This kind of pelvis-to-skull picture is still the best option for those suffering from TMJ, whiplash, and other trauma related injuries, as it has been in practice for hundreds of years.

ADVICE FOR MFR TREATMENT

*W*alking into an unfamiliar office can be nerve wracking, especially when you are there to find a solution to a long term affliction. There are a few ways that you can help combat the stress of this initial visit, and even later visits once you have left. Let's walk through a few techniques that can change your daily life in more ways than you know.

Your body can heal! It is important to know first, that your body has the ability to repair itself. Whatever may have happened that brought you here, you have survived it. Your body is resilient! What we do here is open up your body via the fascial system, in order for your body to do what it is made to do. Even though you may be experiencing pain and discomfort in your body right now, it can and will change.

EXERCISE

Exercise is an important part of maintaining a healthy lifestyle. Our body and mind are connected. If you feel stressed, your entire body feels the impact. Consequently, if your body feels better, so does your mind. Physical activity is important as it produces endorphins, chemicals in the brain that naturally reduce pain, stress, and improve sleep. Initially, it is best to refrain from all current exercise regimes while you are new to authentic Myofascial Release Therapy. The safest thing to do is walking; a brisk 20 to 30 minute walk is safe to do while undergoing this therapy.

MOVEMENT

*O*n occasion, you will feel as though your body wants to move, twitch, or shake during a session. We encourage you to allow this to happen. Movement during treatment is quite natural, as fascia is three-dimensional and our body is made to move.

Restrictions run in a non-linear pattern that will involve movement to release. If you are injured due to trauma, it is likely that the injury occurred when the body was in motion. To fully release the trauma pattern held in the fascial system, "unwinding" is recommended and necessary as part of your treatment.

Unwinding is an enlightened movement that occurs when you feel safe, and can let go of control and allow your subconscious mind to release the pattern of trauma that is trapped within the fascial system. Your therapist is trained to facilitate this with you when you are in a safe place to let go of past trauma and allow your body to heal itself.

POSTURE

*H*aving good posture is important for both your physical and mental health. While good posture helps prevent neck and back pain, it also helps by decreasing stress and preventing fatigue. You are particularly susceptible to fatigue when sitting at a desk or computer for an extended period. It's important to remind yourself to sit up straight and walk with your head up to look and feel your best.

Repetitive activities, falls, surgery, poor posture, and motor vehicle accidents are some of the more common ways our tissue can become restricted. Remember that all the above can affect your posture, and the dehydration of the connective tissue will cause your body to compensate and adjust accordingly.

After a Myofascial Release session you will generally feel more at ease and upright, like a weight has been taken off you. You may feel lighter, even taller due to the pressure release from the fascial system.

EMOTIONS

Your body feels. Your brain thinks. Feelings or emotions are a part of releasing pain and dysfunction in our body. Emotions are felt and expressed with the body, and experienced and labeled in the mind. I encourage patients to be present in your body and notice what you are feeling and experiencing in real time. It is this process that will help you to notice and let go of long-held emotions or patterns of movement that helped create your pain.

THE HEALING CRISIS

*A*s you move through your treatments, you may experience what we call a "healing crisis." This can include mild to intense workout pain, the feeling of emotional chaos, or physical pain.

Myofascial Release is different from other types of body work you may have experienced because it addresses restrictions and habitual patterns deep within the fascial system of the body. You will find that the treatment does not end once you get up off the treatment table. Your fascial system may continue to unravel and release for hours or even days after you leave. This is normal. Continue to tune into your body. You may feel exhilarated, moody and emotional, or anywhere in between.

Most people feel better immediately, although some may feel sore or temporarily stirred up. This is called the Healing Crisis. In other words, you may get worse before you get better. As restrictions are released, your body may be shifting its alignment, so you may feel achy in unfamiliar areas. In rare circumstances, you may experience soreness all over. This may be your body asking for more attention as deeper layers of restrictions are uncovered. Gently stretch these areas. In most cases, soreness will dissipate within a couple of days and then you will feel freer within your body. It's best to drink lots of water. After treatment, it is important to re-hydrate and flush toxins out of areas that were restricted. Healing is not an event. It is a process. Your restrictions did not show up overnight. Myofascial Release is an authentic healing approach that can help you reduce pain, enhance inner tranquility, and improve the quality of your life.

While this may be uncomfortable, it is part of the healing process. Your body has been holding on to a pattern of restriction for a while, and when it is finally released, it is natural to feel it in the form of a discomfort. When you have been out of touch with part of your body due to fascial restriction, what you experience in a healing crisis is more of a "waking up" process. Allowing yourself to feel this is important to the process, as is being gentle with yourself.

HYDRATION

Consuming enough water has many benefits for your health. It is commonly recommended to consume eight 8-ounce glasses of water a day. Water helps you de-stress by providing you with more energy and easing tension. It can also support a healthy weight because when you are hydrated, your body works more efficiently.

The human body is made up of approximately 50-75% water. Drinking water is essential in regulating your body temperature, maintaining joint health, and delivering essential vitamins and minerals. Water is involved in almost every bodily function, from digestion to circulation. It can increase your energy, improve kidney function, and give you healthier skin.

Dehydration, on the other hand, leads to impaired nerve and muscle function caused by the imbalance of sodium and potassium in the body. Brain and muscle function also become impaired, decreasing muscle coordination and hindering athletic performance.

Warning signs and symptoms of dehydration can include headaches, dry mouth, chills, dry skin, excessive thirst, and fatigue. Signs of worsening dehydration are an increase in body temperature and heart rate, confusion, vision disturbances, or difficulty breathing, for which you should seek medical attention.

The American Council on Fitness suggests following this guideline:

1. Drink 17-20 ounces of water two to three hours before the start of exercise.

2. Drink 8 ounces of fluid 20-30 minutes prior to exercise or while warming up.

3. Drink an additional 8 ounces of fluid within 20 minutes after exercising.

While this may seem like a lot, it shows many of us how little water our body is getting compared to what it actually needs. The easiest way to measure your level of hydration is through your urine, which should be almost colorless and odorless. Try to keep drinking water, as no other beverage hydrates the body better than water.

Fascia and connective tissue is made up of 70% water, contributing a huge portion to the body's general hydration. Water is necessary for the fluidity of our fascia as a result of this. Being dehydrated causes us and our fascia to become rigid and inflexible.

When fascia restrictions exist in the tissue, it is like pouring water over a rock: the water is not able to permeate through to reach the cellular level, until the restrictions are released. Trauma, surgery, and inflammation can also dehydrate the fascia and cause our tissue to begin to solidify. Myofascial Release will help restore the hydration of the solidified tissue, and hydration is necessary to return fascia to its normal state of fluidity, once the restrictions are released.

EAT WELL

Constant or frequent stress can cause a spike in appetite and can lead many people to reach for unhealthy foods. It's important to think of your food as fuel and make choices that are good for your body and energy levels. Some healthy choices that help your body to naturally de-stress are blueberries or other foods that contain antioxidants.

SLEEP WELL

*I*t's important to sleep well and to get enough to reduce the effects of stress. Missing out on sleep can cause irritability, drowsiness, and trouble concentrating. Sleep deprivation also leads to increased stress levels, which can cause high blood pressure and the production of stress hormones. This increases your risk for heart attack and stroke. It's important to learn which relaxation techniques work for you to counteract the effects of stress and get quality sleep.

Sleeping with two pillows can cause havoc for your neck, if they don't support your head correctly. Two pillows may tilt your head forwards and prop your head upwards. This puts your head in an unusual position that it will continue to be in for about eight hours. Not just your head, but also your neck, feels that continual pressure. With the head not supported correctly, the neck takes on the role of support while you sleep. That's an abundance of pressure to be on your neck for eight hours!

A helpful rule is to sleep with one pillow. While it takes some adjustment and may feel weird or flat at first, it will make a great difference once you're adjusted to it. One pillow will support your head and allow the body to stay in line, giving your neck a necessary rest.

Reading, checking emails, or playing on your phone before bed. Whichever it is, the same action is applied to all of them. As you unwind in bed doing any of the above, your head is tilted. In this tilted position, your head is no longer being supported by your shoulders, but your neck alone. Your neck compensates for this by tensing its muscles to keep your head where it is. With these muscles tensed, your body is in an unusual position. If you read, check emails or play on your phone for about one hour each night, it's no surprise that your neck is hurting!

Imagine going to bed with two pillows and reading for about an hour. It's easy to see in this scenario how you may be causing your neck to be in pain before your head even hits the pillow! Your neck has been in an uncomfortable position since reading, and you're just going to put it into another unusual position by sleeping on two pillows for eight hours.

Being cognizant of how your body is designed and the ways that we can adjust our habits to accommodate this can make all the difference in the world when it comes to getting good sleep and painless mornings.

MANAGE YOUR TIME

*B*eing busy can be overwhelming. It's important to manage your time well to reduce stress. Prioritizing your tasks and activities can help you use your time well. Utilizing a daily schedule or planner to break everything down helps ensure you don't feel overwhelmed by everyday tasks and deadlines.

HAVE A GOAL

Having a clear and realistic goal for treatment will help you achieve the results you are looking for. While being "pain-free" sounds nice, it is not always realistic, especially within a specific time frame. Having a clear goal in mind to share with your therapist will help you and your therapist achieve success. An example of a clear goal like, "I would like to have no pelvic pain and be able to go for a 5 mile bike ride." is in contrast to an unclear goal such as, "I want to no longer have pain." The more clear you can make your goal, and the more time you put towards achieving it, the greater chances for success with reaching it. Just showing up to your treatment is not enough; a lot goes into self-care, as well.

COMMUNICATION

*C*ommunicate with your therapist regularly during treatment by letting them know what you are feeling. It will greatly help your therapist understand you better and how your body experiences and processes treatment. On occasion, your therapist will ask if you notice anything during or after a session. There is no wrong answer. Everything is valid. Even if your answer is "nothing," you are providing your therapist with valuable information. Benefits of the session may not always be immediately obvious.

PRACTICE RELAXATION

*M*ake room in your schedule for activities that bring you calmness and joy. This time can also be useful for finding which relaxation techniques work best for you. This can include deep breathing, meditation, or progressive muscle relaxation. Adjust your lifestyle accordingly. Small changes, such as less reading time before bed or getting one supportive pillow, will make a difference, easing any neck pain that may be caused at night. Overall, taking a mental break to refocus can be very beneficial.

BREATHING EXERCISES

*B*reathing exercises are well-known for being a quick and effective de-stress method. Breathing exercises can help you relax because they make your body feel like it does when you are already relaxed. "Belly breathing" is simple to learn and very relaxing. Try it anytime you need to relax or relieve stress:

1. Sit or lie flat in a comfortable position.
2. Put one hand on your belly just below your ribs and the other hand on your chest.
3. Take a deep breath in through your nose, and let your belly push your hand out. Your chest should not move.
4. Breathe out through pursed lips, as if you were whistling. Feel the hand on your belly move with your breath, and use it to push all the air out.
5. Do this breathing exercise three to ten times. Take your time with each breath and notice how you feel at the end of the exercise.

STAY CENTERED

Staying centered is a helpful tool in lifelong stress reduction. Mindfulness for stress relief and relaxation can be utilized no matter where you are. The core practices of mindfulness are intention, attention, and attitude. These lead to "reperceiving," which is when mindfulness allows us to dis-identify from thoughts, emotions, and body sensations. We realize that we are not controlled by them and this gives us the ability to see a situation as it really is.

IF INJURED

*I*ce should typically be used for acute or recent injuries, commonly ankle or knee sprains, for the first 72 hours after an injury. The RICE formula for acute injuries is Rest, Ice, Compression, Elevation. Ice will help reduce the swelling that causes pain.

Applying an ice pack or bag of frozen vegetables to an injury should be done for no more than 10 to 15 minutes at a time. While it is okay to have direct exposure to the ice if it is short-term, it is always recommended to apply a layer between the ice and your skin. This could be a simple cloth barrier, like a thin bath towel. It is also helpful to keep the ice moving to avoid frostbite. Using ice on your left shoulder is not advised if you have a heart condition.

The reason that icing an injury should only be done in the short-term and with caution is that when connective tissue becomes cold, it loses much of the elasticity that is needed for healing. The interstitial fluid that fills the small spaces between the structures of your body also thicken, slowing down the processes, as well. When you constrict elasticity and blood vessels, you are restricting the blood supply to the very place that it is needed most, possibly damaging tissue permanently. There is no reason to ice an injury if it has been six or more hours.

On the other hand, heat has the opposite effect of ice, as it causes blood vessels to open, which can stimulate inflammation rather than relieve it. For this reason, heat should be used on chronic conditions for soothing stiff joints, relaxing muscles, relaxing tissue, and to stimulate blood flow to the injured area. Heat is the best option for old injuries or even arthritis. Your heat source can be from a heating pad or even a hot damp towel. You should not use heat after activity or an acute injury because it can cause your swelling to worsen, increasing pain.

Moderation is important to remember for both heat and ice. It is possible to suffer from burns due to excessive use of hot or cold pain remedies. Always remember to remove your heat or ice for at least 15 to 20 minute intervals.

While ice and heat are effective in temporarily reducing the symptoms, it doesn't treat the source of your pain. For treatment that is effective in treating the source of your pain, you should seek physical therapy. Your physical therapist can help you treat the source of your pain and provide you with exercises and strategies to avoid injury in the future.

TAKE CARE OF YOUR FASCIA AT HOME

*I*t is so important for me to empower my patients so they know what to do when their body starts to talk to them with different symptoms. I truly enjoy teaching them how to be more body aware, and follow the feeling, as well as know what they need to do when they feel certain symptoms. I take pride in teaching safe, self-corrections, and gentle Myofascial Release stretches, as well as stability exercises that they should routinely perform without me to keep up the effects of what we do together in their sessions. The treatments in the clinic are always much more lasting when the patient takes their health into their own hands and becomes an active participant, on and off the treatment table.

STRETCHING

I often get asked about stretching. Most people are accustomed to holding a stretch for 20 to 30 seconds. I find that to be far too rushed. When I tell patients this, I am often met with some very surprised faces. People will make excuses; they are too busy to dedicate more time to the simple act of stretching, they feel as if they can't do, and more.

It is mind-boggling to me that some people cannot find even five minutes to spare in order to better themselves. Rushing through life might get you to places faster, but what use is that if you are hurt and broken when you get there? I encourage each and every one of my patients to think of themselves as their most precious possession, and to take care of themselves as such.

This brings us to the many ways that you can practice self-care in the form of MFR at home. Namely, fascial stretching. Facial stretching is one of the more notable hallmarks of MFR therapy, and when properly educated, can be a useful tool to continue your therapy within your own home.

First, it is important to note that the only way to practice MFR at home is to do so with caution and under the care of a therapist. You must approach it knowing that you will need patience, both physically and emotionally, in order to reap benefits from it. It takes a minimum of five minutes in each hold to get down to the ground substance of tissue. Again, we can take the example of an orange. Think of the inner rind, that white, dried out substance that makes up the innermost layer. This substance is similar to the ground substance within the body that is depleted of hydration.

Tissue can become dehydrated for various reasons that have been mentioned previously. When this occurs, you become susceptible to pain and immobility. This means that it is incredibly important to utilize your foam roller to soften, not force, your fascia. Notwithstanding the name of this practice, you do not want to roll your tissue. This action will not allow the connective tissue that you are working on to release naturally and fully. What you do want to do is move the roller over the superficial layer of tissue at the surface.

Think of pulling a rubber band and letting it snap back into place. When you are using your foam roller to push the tissue or perform a hold for less than 90 seconds, you are causing your tissue to do exactly that. When you tense or tighten, you are creating new holding patterns elsewhere in the body. Instead, the goal is to soften the connective tissue and patiently wait to sink into the tool. Listen to your body and adhere to the limits that it places. The key to release is to take the time that you need to learn to listen to your needs, and reflecting that same time in treating it. Once you begin to soften into the ball, or whatever tool you prefer to use, you will never return to stretching the way that you had been before!

PATIENT CARE & TREATMENTS: FOR MY FELLOW THERAPISTS

*W*hen we get used to a mundane routine, one that repeats itself over and over again, for months, and then years, we can start to lose sight of the most important part of the process: why we are doing it in the first place. Eventually our goals become routine. (The American Association for Aesthetic Plastic Surgery, 2019)

Your brain is programmed to go into autopilot mode so that it can become more efficient at the things it thinks you need to do every day. This is a result of biological evolution, a process that allows you to save your thinking power for more important things, like hunting and survival. Unfortunately, when this autopilot mode switches on in something like bedside manner, the patient can be the victim of the mental efficiency.

Many doctors and therapists find themselves seeing patients as just another number on their spreadsheets after many years in the field. These patients are just part of a greater, emotionless day of service and support. Because of this, patient care can fall to the wayside. In fact, I once had an employee of mine confess that their former clinic ran on the motto, "Treat 'em and street 'em."

At the end of the day, patients are still human beings. Patients are people with stories, families, and beating hearts, which means they shouldn't be treated like just another cog in the machine. They are in your care because they are in need, and you are there to provide that. Our duty is to do so in the most caring way possible.

Sometimes a physician, counselor, or therapist doesn't necessarily have to be blunt or rude. They can be dehumanizing in subtler ways. It can be the stripping of a patient's clothing, or the calling of the patient by their condition, as opposed to their name. It can be subjecting a patient to tests and exams they don't understand with doctors they've never met, repeating the same history several times to different people in the same clinic, or talking at them instead of with them.

The truth of the matter is this kind of dehumanizing behavior is so common that there's an entire research center designated to changing it. I have observed countless examples of the above behavior. Although I was not the therapist to the patients I observed being treated this way, I truly felt for them, and wished I could show them how a therapy session could be. Regardless of who I'm treating, with every patient encounter, it is my top priority to make them feel like a person first, and a patient second. I try to connect with them emotionally, and deliver exceptional service so they have a "WOW" experience. Being passionate and determined, as well as humble, is what allows me to prosper.

The good news is, if you're afraid your bedside manner is anything but supportive or respectful, you can change it today. You don't have to allow autopilot to take over your thinking. You can make a decision to change up your routine so that your "autopilot" incorporates kind and protective services.

I make it a point to get treated by a Myofascial Release therapist I met through class every five weeks. That's right, I don't have pain anymore, and I drive an hour, sometimes a little longer, to get treated regularly. Why? Like I mentioned, I don't have pain at this point, but I do a lot of repetitive tasks that tend to cause tissue restrictions. I believe in practicing what I preach, and getting treated is a big part of that. Myofascial Release is truly the healthcare of the future. Getting treated for prevention purposes is how you can truly age gracefully.

As a second benefit, I love to get treated because it reminds me of what a patient may feel like when they are on my treatment tables at

Arancia PT. It's also very important for me to remember to quiet my mind, stay centered within my body, and feel. Feel the techniques fully, listen to my fascial voice as my body is starting to unwind, and stay present. Gently softening and giving my body permission to let go and self-correct is huge. Every time I get treated I return to work feeling invigorated, more centered, and more joyful.

I have had the benefit of working in a variety of different settings before I opened up my own clinic, Arancia PT. Prior to opening up, I worked at a small, but busy outpatient clinic, where I learned some critical business do's and don'ts. I was fortunate to have my own office at this clinic, and did everything in my power to make my patients' journey, from the first phone call with the receptionist all the way to their discharge visit, special and unique. This has allowed me to compile a comprehensive list of ways to stave off this compliancy, that so many others in the medical profession give way to, by being aware of my demeanor and actions.

For my fellow DPT's, and any other health care professional who may stumble across this book, here are some basic guidelines for treating patients with actual care:

1. Always Knock:
    Regardless of how busy your day might be, barging into a room without knocking is always a rude thing. The simple gesture of giving the patient some space and privacy will have them feeling like a human, as opposed to a science experiment.

2. Ask About Names:
    We all have names, and we all want to be called by our names. Asking your patient their name and what they want to be called is a powerful way to acknowledge them as an individual. Even if their name is Alexandra, they might want to be called Allie, Alex, or Alexa. Making

a note of that and remembering it each time will make them feel like a real person in your office.

3. Leave for Changing:

    If the patient needs to strip down for evaluation and treatment purposes, don't just stand there and watch them. Kindly exit the room, wait next to the door, and ask them to signal you back in when they are ready. No one wants to be completely naked in front of a stranger. Also, when it comes time for you to review your evaluation findings, and discuss a plan of care, give them the opportunity to get dressed back up. Standing there while they are half naked and telling them what's going on leaves them in a very vulnerable and uncomfortable position. Leave the room, wait for them to change, and return when they're ready to resume.

4. Validate Concerns:

    You're the medical expert in the room. The patient is probably scared about their current pain or functional limitation, and they want you to reassure them it will be ok. When they tell you about their problems, validate them and explain why. Help the patient further understand the situation at hand. Don't make them feel like they are being over emotional or irrational.

    If you really want to make someone feel special, respond with something like, "Tell me more," instead of shutting down their explanation once you have the information you need. We all want to be heard, seen, and understood. Go out into the world today and make it a point to remember that patients are human beings, just like you and I. You'll find your receptivity and respect as a

Doctor of Physical Therapy, or health care professional, will increase tenfold.

5. Keep Learning:

   Just because you have graduated and obtained a license to treat patients doesn't mean learning should cease. Although some states do not require continuing education credits, it is your responsibility to obtain the most up-to-date treatment knowledge for the benefit of your patients. Your career is about lifelong learning. Fine tune your clinical skills, and even more important, your communication skills.

THE FASCIAL NETWORK: WHAT THERAPISTS OF MYOFASCIAL RELEASE HAVE TO SAY

There is a large network of men and women in America who practice Myofascial Release. Together, we have explored a side of physical therapy that many do not, and as such, trust in one another's expertise. These people have become strongholds of innovation and support in the fight against chronic pain.

Although each therapist practices the same art of healing, no two are the same. You will never walk into my clinic and receive the exact same experience as you would in any other, even if both myself and the other practitioner have studied under the same mentor and offer similar services. This is what makes us so great. We are unique, just as you are. We all have come to this point in our journey through different means, yet still have the capability of bringing relief and peace to our patients.

I have asked colleagues of mine a couple of questions to get their take on their views on Myofascial Release, to highlight the many different therapists you may find along your own path. You will find their practice information above their name. They have graciously trusted me with their stories. I would now like to share them with you.

Maureen McCloskey, MSPT

MFR Expert
BodieMOtion, Rye Brook, NY
BodieMOtionPhysicalTherapy.fullslate.com

*M*aureen and I first met in Key West, FL during an amazing course titled "Quantum Leap" in 2016! Although we met only briefly back then, I truly became inspired by Maureen when she spoke up in a later class where we were discussing patient care and the initial evaluation process.

As she began to describe her encounters with new patients, especially the ones who are new to the Myofascial Release approach, I could literally feel the hairs on my arms stand up. Her passion for this work is incredible, and she, much like myself, can't help but let it spill into more than just the professional workplace.

She spoke about how she loves to educate her patients, family, and friends on the importance of the fascial system. This resonated deeply within me, as many of the clients who come in are not aware of the fascial system and how it can be an overlooked source of underlying trauma, pain, and restriction.

J.P: "How did you learn about the JFB Approach?"

M.M: "About 20 years ago when I worked at a children's rehabilitation hospital, I attended an 'in-service' given by an OT on the JFB Approach. The hospital paid for her to attend the course, and in turn she educated the staff about what she had learned. This therapist and I were both assigned to the same child who had suffered severe burns and received skin grafts to much of his body. All measures of progress had been very slow. The therapist showed me how to perform a 'crossed-hand' technique that she had practiced during the John F. Barnes seminar. She and I worked on the child together using the technique we had just been taught. The results were astonishing, even from that first encounter. The child regained motion in his joints quickly, had markedly reduced pain, and his function improved so that he was able to run around once again.

My next encounter with learning the JFB Approach came ten years later as a patient. Within a 5 year period, I had surgeries to my cervix, a C-section, open exploratory surgery, a large hamartoma (benign tumor) and coccyx resection, bowel obstruction and an inguinal hernia repair. I sought out therapists trained by John F. Barnes to assist in my healing and recovery. I was suffering with urinary incontinence, experiencing painful intercourse, and joint pain. From that first treatment as a patient, I knew it was the missing link in my care, and in health care in general. I knew I was on the road of authentic healing. As a therapist, I also knew that I wanted to learn as much as I could to assist others on their healing journey.

In 2010, as I was being treated regularly, I began taking John F. Barnes seminars. From the very first seminar with John, I knew I was 'home.' I have never looked back. To date, I have taken all of John's seminars, and many of them repeatedly. I look forward to each seminar as a present that I can share with the people I encounter each day: my family, my friends, my patients, and strangers. I continue to get treated regularly, and I am often asked to assist John and the other instructors with seminars."

J.P: "What type of therapy were you practicing prior to MFR? Would you go back to it? And lastly, did you learn anything about fascia in grad school?"

M.M: "Since fascia has been ignored in health care and in my education, I now consider the therapies I learned and used prior to the JFB-MFR

Approach to be, at best, temporary fixes and at times injurious. There is no going back to forcing tissues (fascia) to release.

Fascial releases require gentle, sustained pressure of five minutes or more to occur. There is no going back to trying to 'fix' people. Therapists facilitate healing, but people ultimately heal themselves. There is no going back to strengthening tissues that are restricted and tight. Tight muscles are not strong muscles. There is no going back to treating diagnoses. We treat people and treat what we see/feel second to second. There is no going back to treating based on a protocol. Each person is unique. There is no going back to a symptomatic approach to treating patients. We are not made up of parts functioning independently. We are a whole body and *everything* is connected via the fascial system. Every cell of the body interacts with the fascial system. Every system of the body is affected by the fascial system."

J.P "What impact has MFR had on your life, personally and professionally?"

M.M: "I could not tell my story without sharing how JFB-MFR helped me to help my sister, Sheila, when she was in excruciating pain from stage four appendix cancer. Although my sister was taking very heavy pain medication, she was still too uncomfortable to fall asleep.

One night as I lay beside her, I remembered the little boy with burns and skin grafts whom I helped in the children's hospital alleviate his pain. I put my hands on my sister and used the principles I had been taught years earlier. My sister fell asleep then, and often requested for me to 'do that thing you do with your hands' many times afterwards. It did not cure my sister, but it allowed her to be in less pain when the pain was unbearable. After my sister passed away, my decision to treat others with chronic pain using JFB-MFR became clear. I will always be grateful for John and the work he has developed and shared with the world.

I think the most profound personal impact that JFB-MFR has had on me was releasing past emotional and physical trauma. As my body let go of stored emotions and I felt into areas of my body which were

traumatized, I became more whole. My pain is gone and my incontinence is significantly improved (nerves had been severed during the
surgery). Less than a year and a half after my first JFB-MFR treatment,
I completed my first Ironman Triathlon (2.1 mile swim, 112 mile bike,
26.2 mile run). Without JFB-MFR, this accomplishment would not have
been possible. Everyday I am in awe of this work, however, it is one of
my first experiences treating a patient that I remember as particularly
remarkable.

I was working as an independent contractor for the NYS Early
Intervention program. I made a home visit to an 18 month old child
with developmental delays and an ataxic gait. He tended to hold onto
furniture as he moved for stability. He could not cross an open space in
the living room without falling down. On this particular day, the child
was still sleeping when I arrived. I used several techniques, including
a dural tube release that I had recently learned, before the child woke
up crying and sweating. The mother asked me what happened and I
explained that sometimes it could be a response to treatment, as restrictions are released and the body realigns. I assured her that I had not
injured her son. On the outside I was calm, but on the inside, I admit,
I was a little nervous (even though I had experienced similar reactions
myself during treatment). A few days later, at my next scheduled visit,
I opened the elevator door and the child 'ran' out of the apartment and
down the long hallway into my arms. I will never forget that moment
and his smile. The mother was so grateful and so was I."

**J.P: "What is one piece of advice or wisdom you would share with
anyone interested in learning more about this approach?"**

M.M: "Get treated regularly by a JFB-MFR therapist. 'You can take your
patient as far as you are willing to go yourself,' as John F. Barnes has
said. Many people claim they know MFR, but if it isn't JFB-MFR, it isn't
the real thing. Attend a seminar! Then, repeat. Read John's book *Healing
Ancient Wounds: The Renegade's Wisdom* (2000). Then, reread it."

J.P: "Please share a little bit about your practice and what types of patients you treat. What percentage are Women's Health? How do your patients find you? Are they coming in specifically for Myofascial Release and/or Women's Health?"

M.M: "I opened my practice in 2014 within a yoga/cycling studio. Many of my first patients were athletes from my triathlon crowd, or patrons of the studio who came in for injuries from their particular sport or exercise. However, because fascia affects all other systems, it was quickly realized by all receiving the work that this approach can treat everyone for just about everything. Word spread.

I moved locations after the first year to a dance studio. Here, I see people of all ages and for just about anything you can think of. Word of mouth and John F. Barnes' Therapist Directory are the two most common ways people find me. I also receive referrals from several doctors. Some I have never met, but their patients are walking billboards. Other doctors have been curious and open enough to be treated by me so they also refer to me. I treat all people, but a sampling includes: people post-mastectomy; people with fertility issues; people who have pain with intercourse and incontinence; people with joint and spine pain, looking to avoid surgery and recovering post-surgery; people with bowel dysfunction; people with plantar fasciitis, neuromas, migraines, vertigo, frozen shoulder; athletes recovering from injuries, wanting to prevent injuries, and perform better.

Some people come in specifically for Women's Health issues, especially if they were referred by someone who has been helped with their own issues. But more often, women I see are not even aware that 'Women's Health' treatment exists for their pelvic floor issues. A common expression I hear is: 'I just thought I had to learn to live with it.' When they learn that JFB-MFR is a viable, non-surgical and pharmacological option, many seek out the work for their specific need."

Amy Vander Linden, MSPT

MFR Expert
Moment of Truth Physical Therapy, Phoenix, AZ
Momentoftruthpt.com

I met Amy at a business course a few years ago in Las Vegas, NV. I was in a room surrounded by over 150 physical therapist business owners. I overheard Amy talking about her practice and immediately could tell she was an MFR trained therapist. I went over to her and introduced myself, and we instantly clicked and became good friends. Amy has a practice specializing in Women's Health in Arizona and recently expanded her clinic to incorporate a wellness center. If you are ever in the Phoenix, AZ area, you must stop by her clinic!

J.P: "How did you learn about the JFB approach?"

A.L: "As therapists, we have to do con-ed every year. I had received a flyer advertising Myofascial work with John Barnes. I went to my first course in Sedona, AZ in March 2009."

J.P: " What type of therapy were you practicing prior to diving into MFR?"

A.L: "I was previously doing physical therapy in a wellness center, helping clients become able to do exercises without pain or limitations, as they had when they entered our program. I then branched into home health while taking more MFR classes and growing my private practice."

J.P: "Had you learned about fascia prior to taking an MFR class?"

A.L: "No, not a word about it in school or other continuing education courses I had taken previously."

J.P: "What impact has MFR had on your life, personally and professionally?"

A.L: "MFR has changed everything about my life for the better. MFR helped me learn to trust myself, my instincts, my hands, and truly helped me grow. I learned how to be centered and that has overflowed into all areas of my life. It gave me back the ability to offer true, authentic healing, the reason I went to school in the first place. Embracing the courses and this work gave me a niche that led me to start my own practice. John's courses are even what guided me into Women's Health, and ultimately guided my practice to where it is today.

When you start taking courses they advise getting worked on to continue your own growth and education, but more importantly our own healing. We can only take clients where we are willing to go, so this work has given me more healing, more wholeness, more awareness, and that overflows into all areas of my life. If I shared everything, I'd have to write my own book, but it has definitely impacted my parenting and my marriage. I have two children and they are often a mirror for the good and bad within us. We are inspired to do better because they are watching. We also know that anything left unhealed in us gets passed on to them. Myofascial work, specifically learning to trust myself and embrace FEELING, has changed everything about me for the better. I typically prefer anger to grief, fun over sorrow, and thinking over feeling. That is part of who I am, both from nature and nurture growing up. I have learned how to embrace grief, honor sorrow, feel ALL the feelings, which lets me experience greater joy. This was also a critical piece for me having that ability when walking with my clients, husband or kids through things. Plus, they love getting worked on.

I have clients who have been through unspeakable and unimaginable things, particularly working with pelvic health. Many clients have experienced miscarriages and several assaults. Because of this work, I can hold that space for them. Not because I've been there. Not because I truly understand what they've experienced, but because I've done the work to get clear. I've worked on my own traumas–being raised by a single mother, moving across the country when I was 12, and all the other things that pile on just from living life. We all have layers of physical, emotional, and mental traumas, wounds to our inner child, that need to be healed. I continue getting worked on, taking classes, and facing my own stuff so that I can be with them as they process, can keep them safe for whatever comes up.

True Myofascial Release, in its best form, with a therapist present and aware, a client open and trusting, is pure magic! Every session is new and has tremendous possibility."

J.P: "What is one piece of advice or wisdom you would share with anyone interested in learning more about this approach?"

A.L: "Take a class. With John. Show up. Bring your whole self and find a new level of wholeness you didn't even know was there. There are a lot of amazing courses out there and lots of effective manual techniques. But if you're interested in true authentic healing, the art of touch and fascial connections, there is nothing better than Barnes' Myofascial Release."

J.P: "Please share a little bit about your practice, and what types of patients you treat."

A.L: "My practice is called Moment of Truth Physical Therapy. We specialize in pelvic health. I have a massage therapist and a PTA, and also a customer care specialist. Together, we help women have healthy, active pregnancies, optimal deliveries, and faster recoveries to get back to the activities they love. Using Myofascial Release is at the heart of how we resolve painful restrictions and balance asymmetries, how we help women feel their best throughout their pregnancies, and aid in tissue healing for postpartum recovery. We also address other types of pain and pelvic conditions, but pregnant and postpartum women are the focus at the Moment of Truth Physical Therapy, and Women's Health comprises at least 80% of our practice."

J.P: "How do your patients find you? Are they coming in specifically for MFR?"

A.L: "Some find me on the John Barnes' Myofascial Release Directory. Some find me on Facebook. I try to answer questions or provide resources in several moms groups. Some find us on Google, particularly if they Google MFR near them since there aren't that many of us, even in Phoenix, AZ. My website has two free reports that I offer, as well as exercise videos, blog posts, weekly wellness tips, and my podcast. We try to connect with people through those ways, as well."

Rachel Williams, MSPT

MFR Expert
Riverdale Midtown Physical Therapy, Riverdale, New York
Riverdalemidtownpt.com

I first met Rachel in Ocean City, MD, at my first Women's Health course taught by John Barnes. To be honest, I was terrified at the thought of receiving internal pelvic work, but ultimately knew that it would deepen my understanding of fascial restrictions and pelvic health. It would allow me to dialogue much better with my patients, and be more sensitive to how they may feel and react to the techniques. Rachel was an instant support and mentor to me. We hit it off quickly and have become great friends. Since I first met her in 2015, she has always lent me her ear to listen, allowed me to pick her brain, and given me gentle nudges in the right direction.

J.P: "How did you learn about the JFB approach?"

R. W: "I was working in a traditional OP ortho clinic. One of the massage therapists came back from taking MFR. He was incredulous at all of the 'crazy' things that were going on at the course and told me to go and take it so I could laugh and have a fun weekend."

J:P: "What type of therapy were you practicing prior to MFR?"

R.W: "I was a traditional manual therapist. I included various techniques, such as Mulligan, McKenzie and Maitland."

J.P: "Did you learn anything about fascia in grad school?"

R. W: "Yes! We learned on day one of cadaver anatomy that we needed to remove all of the goopy, glue stuff that was in the way, and literally throw it in the garbage cans on the floor so that we could learn about the important structures."

J.P: "What impact has MFR had on your life, personally and professionally?"

R.W: "It has given me back the patience and ability to tap into and listen to not only my hands, but my intuition. It has allowed me to go from a mechanical, procedural practice, to having a creative, engaging practice at Riverdale Midtown Physical Therapy. It has given me the tools to not only treat and reconcile my own injury, but give my patients the ability to be treated, self-treat, and truly heal from the inside out. It is no longer treating symptoms or diagnoses, but treating humans."

J.P: "What is one piece of advice or wisdom you would share with anyone interested in learning more about this approach?"

R.W: "Get treated and get a 'feel' for what the work is like. Be open to reading and satisfying the underlying science and foundation to the work, then just be. Be present and be available to the wonderful gift you are giving to yourself."

J.P: "Please share a little bit about your practice and what types of patients you treat. What percentage are Women's Health?"

R.W: "I have an outpatient community based practice based in Riverdale, NY. I treat a variety of patients and all 'diagnoses.' I prefer to treat the complex patient and patients with Women's Health involvement. About 25% of my caseload is Women's Health."

J.P: "How do your patients find you? Are they coming in specifically for Myofascial Release and/or Women's Health?"

R.W: "My patients find me mainly through word of mouth. MFR has enabled me to make a name and positive reputation for myself as a practitioner in my community. Additionally, I have been able to establish wonderful referral relations with other practitioners in my community, such as a physicist and an acupuncturist. They see the change that MFR makes and are now confident in referring to my practice as a positive intervention for their patients."

Dr. Abel Rendon, PT, DPT

MFR Expert
Rendon Physical Therapy, Loma Linda, CA
Rendonpt.org

*A*bel and I met at a mastermind course in Orlando, FL. I happened to be next to him in line during the lunch break one day, and after a few minutes of chatting, it didn't take me long to learn that he was also a Barnes' trained therapist. Naturally, we had a great deal to discuss.

J.P: "How did you learn about the JFB approach?"

A.R: "I can still remember the exact moment I heard about JFB-MFR. It was in my sixth year of working as a Physical Therapist. I was working per diem at a local skilled nursing facility, providing physical therapy to a sub-acute facility. It was not my ideal setting to be working in, but the pay was needed and I had to pay bills for my growing family.

I had been working for this company for almost a year and getting by, but slowly I was losing my love for the field of PT due to the mass amounts of limitations that third party payers were giving us, forcing us to become 'billable therapists,' and not focusing on what the patient really needed. I felt more and more like I was losing my drive. In the charting room for therapists, I remember sitting next to a veteran OT who had been practicing for more than 20 years, and I had an overwhelming feeling I needed to reach out and ask her something.

I asked, 'Diana, do you ever feel that the way you used to treat and the way you are forced to treat takes the love out of providing therapy for people?'

She set her notes down, turned to me and said, 'Yes, I do. It's very different than it used to be in the field of rehab.'

I said, 'How do you do it? How are you still so energized about providing high-level therapy with all the constraints they are imposing on us?'

Her response paved the way, she said 'Abel, you need to learn about Myofascial Release from John F. Barnes.'"

J.P: "What type of therapy were you practicing prior to MFR?"

A.R: "Prior to MFR training, I was a very conventional 'by the book' practitioner. I had a variety of different job experiences (i.e. Home Health, Workman's comp, Outpatient Ortho, Inpatient Sub-Acute, Ergonomics, Movement screening, Teaching/Labs, Research Assistant, Researcher). So, I felt I was pretty well-rounded, but I didn't know anything about fascial influence on the human body.

During that time frame, I was splitting my time between Outpatient Orthopedics, Sub-Acute Skilled Nursing Rehab, and teaching labs at the local University for second year Physical Therapy students."

J.P "Did you learn anything about fascia in grad school?"

A.R: "No, well that's not exactly true. In Gross Anatomy, we learned to 'Get rid of all the fascia' because it was in the way of the real important stuff that we had to memorize and visualize."

J.P.: "What impact has MFR had on your life, personally and professionally?"

A.R: "MFR has changed me forever. There was such an inner mental hurricane of distress to go into therapy with a brand new implementation and philosophy on why my patient was hurting the way they reported. It was so complex and yet so simple to start treating perfect strangers.

It forced me to learn how to think of myself as a 'facilitator' versus as an interventionist. The greatest change happened to me when I myself needed MFR due to an accident in which I broke my right collarbone. MFR treatments allowed me to return to work in record time and continue healing with minimal effects.

Slowly, I started implementing MFR into every one of my treatments with patients. Without marketing or budget, people started asking me to treat them privately.... And thus the seed was planted on the potential of opening my own private pay MFR and PT clinic. Rendon Physical Therapy and Myofascial Release, Inc."

J.P: "What is one piece of advice or wisdom you would share with anyone interested in learning more about this approach?"

A.R: "To this date, one of the best pieces of advice I've been given was from a physician who is a very good friend of mine. When I started the MFR journey to dive deep into it and learn everything I could about it, he could tell how excited I was to jump in head first and he said this to me, 'I'm glad you are stepping outside the box to improve your clinical practice, but don't forget to be eclectic.'

Be able to evaluate and use a variety of different ideas, styles, or interventions from a diverse range of sources. It's not that I disregard other forms of intervention from my past school, it's just that MFR is the Gold Standard, and no other modality or manuel treatment comes close to the results that MFR has provided for my patients.

MFR is specialized and unique. Many people claim they do MFR, but it's a pure, organic intervention that should not be confused with objects, scrapers, rollers, cupping, percussing or anything that is non-organic which claims MFR."

J.P: "Please share a little bit about your practice and what types of patients you treat. What percentage are Women's Health?"

A.R: "My practice is 100% MFR based. Currently, we offer Myofascial Physical Therapy and Myofascial Massage for our patients. My patient age range is pretty large, 12-72 years of age. My common age group is 35-55 year old females and men who have chronic pain, limiting their quality of life and function.

We offer a treatment intervention that will allow them to leave the dependency of pain pills, injections, or even avoid surgery all together.

Lumbo-pelvic issues are my greatest number of complaints, and it entails about 60-75% of all my patients. Neck pain, shoulder pain, and foot pain round out the other main categories of patients."

J.P: "How do your patients find you? Are they coming in specifically for MFR?"

A.R: "Patients find us on social media (Instagram @rendonpt, Facebook @ Rendon Physical Therapy, Inc.), Google search for Myofascial Release and myofascial pain, our website (rendonpt.org), through our monthly newspaper article that circulates to six different cities around our clinic, farmers market, local gym promotional sites, and the best source of them all, organic word of mouth referrals from past patients.

And yes, for the most part, the majority of the patients come directly seeking MFR. However, due to its limited base of information to the general public, I'm often the first practitioner that describes this process to a new patient who comes in for a discovery visit or consult."

CATHERINE SLIMAN, OTR/L, LMT

MFR Expert
Integrative Kids and Adults, LLC
Integrativekids.com

*W*hen I think of pediatrics, I think of Catherine Sliman. As an Occupational Therapist, my respect for her is great; as a person, it is greater. We met in Pennsylvania in 2016, when I was a student and she was a patient at the Malvern Sanctuary. I was going through my Skill Enhancement Seminar. This is a course to sharpen and expand your skill-set by getting to work in one of John Barnes' clinics as a student therapist. You observe, treat, and get treated during a week long experience. The next time I saw Catherine was at my MFR III course in Sedona, AZ in 2017, where we were both therapists. She has some interesting insight on what it means to treat our youngest patients.

J.P: "How did you learn about the JFB-MFR Approach?"

C.S: " My road to MFR was a winding and an interesting one! I began college as a Pharmacy major, and while I truly loved everything I was learning (science geek!), I did not connect fully to that model of healthcare. At first, we learned about the amazing ability the body has to heal itself, and then we learned how to interfere with that process via medication, which caused side effects. We then had to problem solve how to address those side effects... with more medication, and of course, more side effects. And on and on. It seemed crazy to me that there was no focus on the cause of the symptoms!!

In addition, while working as a Pharmacy Technician, I also saw the beginnings of the opioid epidemic. I saw mothers walk into the store with young children, high as a kite, asking for their narcotic refills. And receive 100 more pills. Always an advocate for children, even at 20 years old, I was horrified. I was ready to call Protective Youth Services, and the Pharmacist filled the script. I knew that day, if that was what was expected of me, I could not be a Pharmacist. So after three years and a very high GPA, I left.

I went to massage therapy school as I figured out my next steps, and it was there that I was introduced to fascia. Dr. Barry Gillepsie came into my class to demonstrate his work, which is derived from his experience with cranial osteopaths, as well as with John F. Barnes Myofascial Release. I was immediately mesmerized and knew that this was what I was looking for: truly helping people by addressing the *cause* of their symptoms!

I continued to study under Dr. Gillespie since that day in 2000, as well as studying with John Barnes, beginning in 2009. I became an Occupational Therapist through Thomas Jefferson University in order to gain greater knowledge about child development and to incorporate fascial work with this population, in which it is so crucially needed! Children become restricted in utero and through the birth process, and this work is so important for successful feeding, overall comfort, and optimal development. I cannot imagine a more rewarding career than helping infants and children thrive, as well as helping to prevent unnecessary and invasive surgeries."

J.P: "What part of Myofascial Release resonates the most for you?"

C.S: "Seeing and hearing about the results in the children I have treated are my greatest rewards. A child with cerebral palsy who could finally dress himself; children with plagiocephaly who avoid helmets and leave with round heads and cranial facial symmetry; torticollis addressed without forceful stretching and superficial results; a child with craniosynostosis who avoided very invasive surgery to her skull, had no obvious head shape differences, and thrived cognitively; and countless babies who have had difficulty with breastfeeding, reflux, constipation, tongue-tie, and more becoming more comfortable in their bodies, learning how to manage the feeding process, and improving the bond with their mothers and families."

J.P "Did you learn anything about fascia in grad school?"

C.S: "During OT school, I would ask many questions about fascia and the craniosacral system, especially pertaining to the conditions we were studying. These questions were always disregarded and blown over. And it was obvious to me that the teaching staff had very little familiarity with these modalities and their relevance to what we were learning. As a new OT, I began to incorporate MFR into my sessions with children in the preschools. I would get strange looks from fellow OTs and PTs, but no one asked what I was doing. After a while, a couple of PTs began asking and I told them proudly, JFB-MFR. One very seasoned PT said to me, 'Oh that is hocus pocus!! My teachers in school said so.' I laughed and kept on treating the way I knew best, with MFR.

Fast forward a few years later, after I opened my private practice, I was still doing some hours at the preschool when this same PT came up to me and said, 'I have a child for you; he could totally use some Myofascial Release.' I was floored! Right then I knew, there had been a turning point and MFR was starting to slowly but surely get the respect it deserves. I saw this turn happen as more and more colleagues began to refer children to me, and even more impressively, they also began to bring their own children to me, as well. I was really happy to see the openness that these professions were beginning to foster, and to literally see the word spread and respect gained for MFR. I opened my practice with the expectation of having one or two clients to start and then advertising and marketing. I was so busy the minute I put my website on the internet, it was overwhelming! It is an exciting time for this work and I am so glad to be able to provide this service, as well as to receive it!"

J.P: "What impact has MFR had on your life, personally and professionally?"

C.S: "I have had some physical and emotional traumas in my life. Besides being born. Ha! I had a very tumultuous childhood, followed by the death of my mother at age 20, and then my father's death nine months later. I was in a major car accident, a skydiving incident, and had a severe concussion all within a couple of years from that.

I was in major pain and had chronic fatigue, not being able to get out of bed 3-4 times a week sometimes. I struggled with endurance, headaches, executive functioning, and memory issues. My body had had enough. I went to physical medicine doctors and neurologists and was recommended to stay sedentary, take aspirin for the rest of my life, and take a little vitamin B. These were not the answers. Receiving MFR was the answer and the only reason I am a functioning human today!"

J.P: "What has MFR done for you, professionally and personally?"

C.S: "MFR has not only opened such an amazing career for me, but has also changed me so much personally. Through releasing my own restrictions, I have learned to be more my authentic self. I have less fear in life and less anxiety about the future. My relationships are stronger and I am able to stick up for myself, rather than always putting others first to my own detriment. I have learned to love myself finally and to love others more fully.

I am so grateful for this work. To know this work, to receive this work, and to practice this work daily. To touch the lives of children and their parents...to make their lives a little easier, a little more joyful, a lot less stressful. To enjoy my own life and to believe I am deserving of it. Nothing feels better."

J.P: "What is one piece of advice or wisdom you would share with anyone interested in learning more about this approach?"

C.S: "My advice to anyone wishing to learn more about this work is to attend a seminar! The Healing Seminar is such a powerful experience and such a privilege. Three days of treatment and learning about MFR (and from John Barnes himself!) is such an invaluable experience, whether you're a seasoned therapist or a patient.

Get treated! Find a therapist to which you feel a connection. I have been to therapists ranging from novice to expert, and sometimes no amount of classes can teach connection. And each connection is unique. One therapist who may be a great fit for you, may not be for your neighbor. If you can trust your therapist, relax, and feel comfortable, more magic can happen! Expert level does not necessarily mean the one for you.

It took me a very long time to read *Healing Ancient Wounds: The Renegade's Wisdom* (2000) by John Barnes. So long that I will not say it here. But it is an amazing resource to learn about this approach. Meditation, yoga, being in nature- any way in which you can get into your body is very helpful. I began my journey with this work thinking it was all just physical. Learning the energetic piece- how to ground myself, maintain my energy, and create boundaries, as well as how to connect to a higher energy- helped me both in giving and receiving the work.

Have fun!! It is easy to feel like you are doing it wrong or don't know enough when learning something new, whether a patient or a therapist. Why didn't I do this sooner? Why did I waste so much time and money with XYZ? Am I supposed to do it this way or that way? Relax! The more relaxed you are, the more you are in your body (see above), and the more effective you can be. Be gentle with yourself and just *feel*."

J.P: "Please share a little bit about your practice and what types of patients you treat. What percentage are Women's Health?"

C.S: "My practice is located in Philadelphia, PA, and has three locations: Center City, South Philadelphia, and Havertown. I treat mostly infants with torticollis, tongue-tie, reflux, plagiocephaly, and breastfeeding issues. I also treat women who are postpartum and other adults with concussions. My referrals come mostly from lactation consultants, pediatricians, physicians, chiropractors, physical therapists, and word of mouth from other clients. I am also listed on the MFR Directory."

Dr. Aaron LeBauer, PT, DPT

MFR Expert
LeBauerpt.com
AaronLeBauer.com

*A*aron Lebauer is a Doctor of Physical Therapy and yoga teacher in Greensboro, NC. Though I have not had the pleasure of making his acquaintance in person, his reputation has preceded him. His experience with JFB Myofascial Release is unrivaled, and his expertise is highly respected. I was ecstatic to receive his insight on what makes this approach so special, and how it has impacted him and his practice.

JP: "How did you learn about the JFB approach?"

AL: "One of my classmates from massage therapy school got a job working with a therapist who used John Barnes MFR techniques, as well as craniosacral techniques. When she treated me I immediately thought this was something great, and that there was something more to what we were learning in massage school. I saw a brochure and attended my first seminar with John Barnes in 2000. Immediately my patients started telling me, 'Wow, you're the first person that's ever touched me, or that's ever been able to help me feel less pain, move better, be more active.'"

J.P: "What type of therapy were you practicing prior to MFR? Would you go back to it? Why or why not?"

AL: "Before MFR, I was studying massage therapy and health education, so deep tissue massage and Shiatsu massage, as well as trigger point therapy. Since then, I've gone back to school to become a Doctor of Physical Therapy, graduating in 2008. Now, I'm combining physical therapy and MFR."

JP: "Did you learn anything about fascia in grad school?"

AL: "A little bit in anatomy class, but we didn't learn about the role of fascia in pain and injuries, and problems like that."

JP: "What impact has MFR had on your life, personally and professionally? Please share a personal and/or professional story."

AL: "MFR has had a significant impact on me, personally and professionally. First off, the network of MFR practitioners has been very supportive of me. Professionally, it's helped me build a practice and a clinical style that gives people results when they can't get results anywhere else. I used to race bicycles, and one year my neck really hurt. Every time I was out training, my neck would lock up and I couldn't get in the bike riding position; I could really only ride sitting up. It was terrible, and it was limiting my treatments. I went to see my local MFR therapist; I actually had to travel quite a bit to see them. We did some rebounding and some MFR and it really helped change the way I felt. Then, I started using a therapy self-care ball to work on the thoracic extension in my back. The combination of those two things really helped me take the problem I was having in my neck and make it so it wasn't as problematic anymore."

JP: "What is one piece of advice or wisdom you would share with anyone interested in learning more about this approach?"

A.L: "Be open to feeling something different. Be open to experiencing it in your body first, and be open to your patient's feelings and/or them experiencing something that you don't even understand, and that's ok. A lot of bodywork, there's a transference of energy, and that's not taught in PT school, and patients will get it, and you'll start to hear it more and more, because what you're able to do is connect more with the soft tissue. The soft tissue dysfunction is something that is more left out of PT school than even just learning about fascia. They just didn't really address soft tissue, and this is an amazing way to address the soft tissue."

JP: "Please share a little bit about your practice and what types of patients you treat. What percentage are Women's Health?"

A.L: "At LeBauer Physical Therapy, we treat active people who want to stay fit, healthy, and mobile without pain meds, injections, or surgery. We are not a Women's Health practice, however, a lot of women who come in with back pain, hip pain, pelvic pain, hamstring tightness, leg problems, shoulder stuff, we find secondarily that they have a pelvic floor dysfunction, a breathing dysfunction or some other issue that goes along with it that's driving the problem they currently have. So, as soon as we start to address that, they get better faster. We refer out for internal work, but we can address the tissue and pelvic floor problems externally with MFR and breathing, etc, and get some amazing results."

J.P: "How do your patients find you? Are they coming in specifically for Myofascial Release and/or Women's Health?"

A.L: "Our patients find us specifically because of our word of mouth strategies, our online email marketing, and Google search. They are not coming specifically to see us for MFR or Women's Health issues; they are coming to see us to solve a problem with which, in order to solve their problem, we use our techniques and skills to do so, and it's an amazing way to give people information. If you're interested in trying Myofascial Release, go get treated, go to one of John's seminars, connect with other people who are doing it as well, and then share your experience!"

Lyn. A. Lunn, OT

Advanced MFR Therapist
Align Therapeutics, LLC, Madison, CT
alignmfr.com

I met Occupational Therapist, Lyn Lunn, at my first skill enhancement seminar at the John Barnes' clinic, The Sanctuary. Together,
we spent our time there shadowing John Barnes as he treated patients in the morning. Midday we received treatments together, followed
by more patient observations. By the second day at The Sanctuary, we
were allowed to assist in treatments under the guidance of John Barnes
himself. She is a gifted therapist and wonderful friend. This is her story.

J.P: "How did you learn about the JFB approach?"

LL: "In 1991, I was a Sophomore college student at the University of
New Hampshire. I had changed my major two times already, starting
with Journalism (I was going to write for a newspaper in Boston) and
then onto Medical Technology (I was going to cure cancer in a lab).
Fortunately, neither of those would actually happen, as the universe
had other plans. My work-study job was at the UNH Child Study and
Development Center– a daycare facility serving children of faculty and
community families. It also supported the Child Study students who
could study child behavior from behind the two-way mirrored windows.
A woman approached me one afternoon, while picking up her children.
She asked me a bit about what I was doing, made some observations

about my skills in interacting with the toddlers, and then stated, 'You are an Occupational Therapist.' I said, 'A what?' I had no idea what she was talking about. She was a Faculty Professor in Pediatric OT at the University, and after meeting in her office the next few days, my life changed. I switched my major, again, and the rest is history. I worked in Pediatrics for the first nine years of my career in acute care and out-patient settings, and then transitioned to adults and geriatrics in skilled nursing facility settings. I loved working with kids, but then I found out, I loved working with adults and older people. As it turns out, I learned that I just basically love working with people, both big and small, and helping them heal.

A JFB Myofascial Release seminar brochure crossed my countertop in 2012. I finally had the opportunity to attend a three-course series in 2014. I have always been drawn to a hands-on approach to facilitating movement and function with all of my patients, both adults and children. MFR seemed like a natural progression of my skills. It felt 'right.' You might think that Occupational Therapy and Myofascial Release is an odd combination. Honestly, I wasn't sure how this would fit into my practice model, especially when most of the people attending the seminars were Licensed Massage Therapists or Physical Therapists. Now I understand it's an absolutely perfect combination. Occupational Therapy (the use of 'occupation' or the patients' 'roles in life' as the therapeutic direction of the treatment) is, by nature, an incredibly holistic practice. It looks at the ENTIRE person– first identifying their roles and occupations (teacher, father, driver, plumber, student, soccer player, etc.), then identifying what impairments are preventing this person from physically and emotionally performing that role.

In my current practice, very often that impairment is pain. So, a mother might come in and she DOESN'T say, 'I want to gain increased flexibility in my spine, increased stability in my legs and improved upper body posture with good freedom of movement.' Instead she might say, 'I want to be able to bend over and pick up my baby and breastfeed him without excruciating pain.' The OT in me looks at her 'occupation': mother/caregiver, etc., and then identifies the problems: impaired postural alignment, muscle imbalances, and soft tissue restrictions preventing her from using her body functionally. Myofascial Release engages the WHOLE body. It also integrates the emotional piece of healing, the part that Western Medicine appears to neglect.

During my first MFR seminar series I learned what was really the tip of the iceberg. Energy and the fascial system were revealed. I began to see and feel things that I never had before. While learning a technique with another therapist, I could feel waves of energy flowing from her. It was unnerving and a little overwhelming at first. I had so many questions! I had been travelling by train in and out of NYC for the seminars. When returning home one evening, I was in a stall in a bathroom at Grand Central station. Glamorous, I know! I had closed the door and was hanging up my backpack when I felt this incredible vibration. I looked down. Was it coming from the floor? I actually reached down to see if I could feel the source. Then I saw them. Little sparkling light energies all around me. As I moved my hands around, I finally realized– they were coming from ME. WHAT??? I spent the rest of the train ride home playing with a ball of energy between my hands– pulling my hands apart and pushing them back together– letting the ball of energy expand and contract between my hands. I laughed out loud because I thought if anyone actually saw me doing this, they would think I was crazy.

My experience the next day was even more profound. It was day seven of a nine day series. I woke up early, and again, caught the train. On my way in, I was filled with a profound sense of peace. An incredible sense of calm. As I left the train and went into the crowds of people scurrying into the city through the subway tunnels and along sidewalks… I began to feel love. Not the kind of feeling, like, 'hey, I love this great cup of coffee!' But the kind of love that you cannot imagine. The kind of love that makes you feel like no matter what happens in your life, you will be absolutely fine. Absolutely no fear. Not only did I feel this internally, but it was flowing out of me. Every single living thing that I saw, I felt an overwhelming sense of love for. Whether it was the little black dog in the subway, or the guy handing out the newspaper at the base of the stairs– I *loved* them. Every. Single. Thing. Then I started to test myself– could I love the person who had hurt me, that I was furious with? *Yes*! Did I love the person sitting next to me in class–*Yes*! I felt like I finally understood that the universe is made of energy, interconnectedness, and *love*. We are energy. I caught a glimpse of something incredibly powerful, and it served to inspire me to continue learning, studying, and growing in the practice of MFR.

About a month after that first MFR series, my daughter Nina, then 16 years old, approached me with a problem. She was having a very difficult time in her self-defense class in high school in the 'choking unit.' She could not stand to be touched on her neck. I said, 'Let's try something.' She sat on a small stool in the kitchen, and I rested my left hand on her head and my right hand on her sternum– with my thumb and index finger lightly resting on her clavicles. This was an approach I had learned in the first Myofascial Unwinding class– the second class in the NYC series. She immediately said she felt pressure on her throat. I asked her, 'What does that feel like?'

'Like your hands are pressing on my chest and closing around my throat,' she replied. 'Let go, I won't let you fall.' She oscillated subtly back and forth, heat pouring off the top of her head. Then, suddenly, she started to cough loudly and repeatedly.

'Let it out,' I said. 'I just did... I feel nauseous– can I sit on the floor?' she asked. I continued to support her in the same way- she started holding her knees with her hands, then her legs extended, hands on her lap. She stayed there for a long time with her eyes closed. I kept my hands lightly on her. Suddenly, she reached out and braced herself with her left hand. She became still, then relaxed, and I helped her gradually rest back onto the floor. She then abruptly 'woke up.'

She said she felt very confused; her abdomen, face and throat hurt. She started coughing more. I asked her how long she was on the floor– she replied, 'A few seconds, then I passed out and woke up.' Her brothers were there– at that time Josh was 14 and Andrew was 10. Josh and I estimated that she was sitting on the floor for at least 10 to 15 minutes before 'falling' back. We asked her about what she had been feeling and she reported that she felt like she was having trouble with her oxygen and like she couldn't breathe. She coughed for about 10 more minutes (note that she was not sick at all when this took place), she felt cold and clammy, and slightly dizzy.

We talked a little more about the experience and I started educating my children about the fascial system, its ability to hold memories and injuries, and just how powerful our own energy is. Josh thought all of this was 'very cool' and told me to 'put me to sleep too!' Haha. Processing this experience later, I have realized that what Nina experienced was likely related to her birth. The umbilical cord was wrapped twice around her neck in utero. Of course, we didn't realize this until the time of her delivery and her heart rate dropped severely with every contraction. She was stuck in the birth canal for a long time. Her fascial system still held onto that experience. Myofascial Release Treatment helped her to release restrictions and process it. She is an incredible young woman now and continues to do her own self-treatment on her neck and jaw. She is still a big fan of MFR.

A little further along in my training in 2016, I traveled to The Sanctuary in Malvern (John's East Coast healing facility), to complete my Skill Enhancement Seminar. I had the wonderful opportunity to meet Jess Papa, the author of this book! It was wonderful to learn alongside someone who was also passionate about the work. We would begin the days early and stay as late as possible, treating and soaking up every ounce of learning that we could in those five days. We were fortunate to treat with, and learn from, incredibly skilled therapists. Most importantly, we had the opportunity to learn directly from John F. Barnes. We witnessed a lot of brave healing during that week. The Sanctuary in Malvern, PA, and Therapy on the Rocks in Sedona, AZ, are very special places. We have remained in touch ever since. I am so inspired by the work that Jess is doing at her practice. I'm extremely grateful that we had the good fortune to meet accidentally in Pennsylvania that week. But really, was it an accident?"

J.P: "What part of Myofascial Release resonates the most for you?"

L.L: "Myofascial Release has connected me energetically to my clients and the world around me. It has shown me what the body is capable of. It has accelerated my practice skills and fueled my inner fire for discovery and detective work! Assessing the body, identifying restrictions, and using your hands to feel deeply into the body for the fine layers of fascial tension is a completely unique way to utilize my therapeutic skills every day. It has amazed me. It has challenged me. Most importantly, it has inspired me to be as holistic and authentic as possible. I've learned to listen to the wisdom of my own body and tune 'in,' not 'out.' I strive to pass that on to my clients. I have my own private practice and treatment studio in Madison, CT. I see adults and adolescents for a variety of reasons– the majority come to solve acute or chronic pain issues (back pain, neck pain, headaches, etc.), scar tissue restrictions, postural alignment, and stress/anxiety/trauma. There are others though, that although I may not be treating them for a Women's Health issue as their primary concern, they find that as their pelvic alignment improves, their digestion improves or even report that intercourse is not painful anymore. A client recently sent me a picture of her legs in the mirror. She was surprised that she no longer has to take her pants to the tailor to hem one side- her legs are now even since her pelvis is level. One of my goals as a practitioner is to develop my skills with a greater focus on Women's Health treatment. I feel that this is a HUGE need in our community. There appears to be such a lack of awareness regarding the effects of pregnancy/delivery/scar tissue restrictions from C-sections or episiotomies, etc. on the pelvis and the whole body– the list goes on!"

J.P: "What are you most excited about as we see more and more innovations in Myofascial Release?"

L.L: "I'm very excited to be part of this wave of awareness of John F. Barnes Myofascial Release. More people are searching for a natural and holistic way to improve their health. Most of my clients find me by word of mouth, through a Google search, or through the JFB Myofascial Release Therapist Directory. I'm currently an Advanced Level Therapist with an ongoing passion to learn more. I love problem-solving and educating people who reach out to me about how JFB-MFR could potentially help them with their specific concerns."

J.P: "What kind of advice would you give someone interested in Myofascial Release?"

L.L: "If you are considering learning more about JFB-MFR, I say, pick up the phone or send a quick email to any trained therapist. You have absolutely nothing to lose by asking some questions. You might learn something that could help you in that moment or you might be inspired to try MFR. Either way, you will have learned something new!"

Justine Calderwood, MSPT

Advanced MFR Therapist
The Healing Spot: Woodland Park, Colorado
Healingspotpt.com

*J*ustine and I met in a rather unexpected way- the new age platform of Instagram! She had initially reached out to me via Instagram and mentioned she had been following my practice, Arancia PT, for some time.

We connected instantly, as we had both found peace and passion in Myofascial Release. Justine is a Birth Healing Specialist and has a practice in Colorado that focuses on treating women by helping them have smooth deliveries and complete recovery postpartum.

J.P: "How did you learn about the JFB-MFR approach?"

J.C: "I learned about JFB Myofascial Release through mailings I received from John F. Barnes, advertising continuing education. I thought the brochures were interesting and they caught my attention, but I just recycled them. I thought the claims I read about in the brochures were too good to be true, but I was always intrigued by the 'Therapy for the Therapist' and secretly wondered if maybe MFR could help me. I didn't think there was anyway I could ever go to Arizona or Pennsylvania to do a 'Therapy for the Therapist' intensive program, but it planted a seed and perhaps gave me a little hope (and insight that maybe I wasn't the only physical therapist around that was suffering with my own pain!).

I had been suffering from chronic daily headaches since my early 20s and nothing up until that point had given me relief. I tried a lot of things: medication (over-the-counter, neurological meds, pain pills, and anxiety medication, which I didn't even think I had!!), dental work that claimed to realign my bite, physical therapy, exercise, and even Botox injections. I gave up hope that anything would help me and I stopped telling my healthcare providers that I had headaches. By some miracle I saved up the money to take MFR 1, and arranged to leave my small children for the weekend so I could see if John Barnes' brochure could possibly be true.

I was not disappointed, and after taking that first seminar in 2013, I was hooked. It was the only thing up until that point that started to shift my pain and really get to the root cause of it."

J.P: "What type of therapy were you practicing prior to MFR?"

J.C: "Up until I took my first MFR seminar in 2013, I was practicing traditional outpatient physical therapy, doing Maitland joint mobilizations, passive stretching, exercise, and teaching my patients about their bodies in the only way I had been taught. I felt ill-equipped to treat anyone with chronic pain and a diagnosis of fibromyalgia completely put me off because I really didn't have much in my bag of PT tricks that I felt could help in any significant way. I felt like a hypocrite because here I was, dealing with chronic pain that I couldn't even figure out for myself, how was I going to help anyone else?"

J.P: What impact has MFR had on your life, personally and professionally?

J.C: "Oh wow, the impact that MFR has had on my life personally and professionally is PROFOUND! For starters, it's the only modality or approach to healing that has actually made my chronic, constant, daily headaches lessen in intensity. I wish I could say that I'm 100% pain-free, even after six years of self-care and MFR sessions, but the intensity has lessened considerably and my quality of life has improved. I used to be so negative and couldn't take a compliment, and certainly couldn't take any criticism, because I was so afraid and judgmental of myself.

I was going through the motions of life, but not really enjoying life at all. I had a lot of anger from my childhood, and lots of old wounds that I didn't really even know were impacting my daily life and my ability to be present in my closest relationships. I had two small children that I wasn't enjoying and whom would often make me feel stressed out and anxious.

I felt unworthy, unlovable, shameful, and anxious most of the time. I didn't like being alone or idle, so I stretched myself to the max and kept myself busy with work, volunteer work, and my children's activities. Looking back, it was my way of avoiding the underlying healing work I needed to face.

After I took MFR 1, my headaches actually got worse for a period of time. I started having ocular migraines, which affected my vision and made it hard to work at times. My physician urged me to go to a different neurologist and get things checked out. After the neurologist took a quick peek at my neck and head, he sat me down and asked me questions about my marriage, my children, and eventually about my childhood. I broke down crying at the mention of my childhood. That was the breakthrough I needed, though. The neurologist referred me to a psychologist, and that started me on a path of opening up to the emotional healing I needed to really get better. During that time, I sought out MFR treatments from a therapist in a neighboring state (the closest MFR therapist was a three-hour drive one way for me), but I got myself to her for some back-to-back sessions so I could see for myself if I could get the relief I desperately needed. Luckily, my psychologist was open to learning about MFR so he could best help me. I started practicing what I had been taught in MFR 1 with my own patients and soon it was apparent that this approach to therapy was different than anything I had learned prior. I became a believer, and for the first time in years, I actually had a glimmer of hope!

Shortly after I started counseling and diving deeper into Myofascial Release, I had a major Healing Crisis. I ended up admitting myself to the hospital for depression and anxiety because I suddenly found myself scared to drive, scared to go to work, lost interest in my life and things that used to bring me joy, and I was having increasing difficulty sleeping and concentrating. I didn't really know what to do, so my psychologist recommended I admit myself to the hospital. While there, I met a psychiatrist who helped me with mood stabilizing medications, which I know I needed at the time.

After things settled down, my psychiatrist urged me to continue with my MFR training. By the time I took Unwinding and MFR in August 2014, five months had passed since my hospitalization. With my psychiatrist's cell phone number in hand, I set off to Chicago for a seven day solo trip to learn more from John F. Barnes. Fast forward five years and I'm off all medications and living life to the fullest. I regularly challenge myself to examine my beliefs, feel my feelings even when they're uncomfortable, forgive others, seek joy, savor the time with my children and husband, and live my life on purpose and with intention.

Personally, MFR gave me a better life with the ability to forgive my past and move forward. It helped me walk away from some toxic relationships in my life, to set boundaries with other relationships, to find my voice, and to feel like a strong and confident woman who is now a healthy role model for her daughters.

Professionally, MFR helped me find the courage to help others on a profound and deep level by opening up my own private practice in physical therapy. I now have the ability to treat patients in a way that I feel good about, with longer sessions, deeper relationships, higher quality of care and for whatever is needed, instead of being limited by my employer or insurance companies. I now feel more self-confident in my abilities as a therapist and I regularly get texts or emails from patients who share about their breakthroughs, their healing, and how much they're able to enjoy life. It brings me so much joy to have a front row seat to others healing. I feel like I'm living my purpose in life.

Oh, and yeah ...in case you're wondering, I DID get to a 'Therapy for the Therapist' intensive program. It happened in 2017. It was a dream come true! I savored every minute of it, remembering that just four short years earlier I thought I'd never be able to do it. And the coolest thing ever about it was that in 2017 I was self-employed and went on my company's expense. So, in a way, I was getting paid to get treated; it brought me to tears when I realized the connection."

J.P: "What is one piece of advice or wisdom you would share with anyone interested in learning more about this approach?"

J.C: "Go for it! Don't listen to the lies that you may tell yourself: that you can't afford it, that you can't travel to the seminars, that you don't have the time or money, or that maybe the claims are too good to be true. If your heart has brought you to this point where you're even considering learning Myofascial Release, I say LISTEN TO YOUR HEART!

It's more than a modality. It's more than a set of techniques. It's a way of life. It's profound healing that will impact every aspect of your life, if you're willing to jump in; not only for you, but for those around you. If you're a therapist, you'll be able to help others on a deeper level than you've ever imagined...if you're willing.

John F. Barnes teaches his therapists that, 'You can only take your patients as far as you're willing to go.' Don't be disillusioned that you'll be able to take MFR classes simply to help others. The only way you'll help others is by first doing your own healing work (or doing your healing work alongside your clients/patients)."

J.P: "Please share a little bit about your practice and what types of patients you treat. What percentage are Women's Health?"

J.C: "I own a 100% cash based physical therapy practice, which means I'm out-of-network with all insurances and patients pay me directly for their sessions. They can submit claims directly to their insurance company, if they choose, and I provide the paperwork they need. I specialize in treating women and men with chronic pain. Chronic pain can be complex, and it's through my own healing journey and my insatiable desire to learn more, that I have a burning desire to heal others who suffer from chronic pain. I remember what it was like to lose hope and to not have the answers or guidance that I needed.

While treating people with chronic pain, I soon discovered that some people had lingering back and hip pain (and even migraines and headaches) that I couldn't quite help them resolve. That's what led me to take John F. Barnes' Women's Health Seminar so I could assess and treat the pelvic floor. I was unsure if I wanted to do Women's Health physical therapy, and in fact it took me about two years to build up the courage to attend that seminar. I went with an open mind that, at the very least, I would perhaps get a little more healing for myself. I left that class with a deeper desire to help more women heal on a deeper level.

Within the past year I have transitioned to seeing 95% women, with a few male chronic pain patients on my schedule here and there. I became a Certified Birth Healing Specialist through the Institute for Birth Healing, which gave me a deeper understanding of Women's Health issues. I use Myofascial Release as the foundation for everything I do as a physical therapist, including teaching patients exercises and stretches, and anything I learn I frame it within the context of what John F. Barnes has taught me about fascia and the three-dimensional fascial network."

J.P: "How do your patients find you? Are they coming in specifically for Myofascial Release and/or Women's Health?"

J.C: "My patients find me through Google (Google Reviews are very helpful), are referred to me from their friends and loved ones (past patients of my mine), on social media (I've built a following on Facebook and Instagram where I educate about MFR, fascia and the whole body approach to healing), or are referred by my power partners (mostly midwives and a lactation consultant that I network with regularly).

I have a listing on the MFR Directory, but people rarely find me there. Some of my patients specifically ask for Myofascial Release, but most of them just want to get better and want to know I can help them.

My female patients are coming specifically for Women's Health issues, such as pelvic organ prolapse, diastasis recti, breastfeeding concerns, incontinence, pain during sex, pelvic pain due to childbirth, infertility concerns, pregnancy related pain, and preparation for a natural childbirth. 85% of my women patients are either pregnant or in early postpartum recovery."

SHANNON REGNER, MSPT, PRPC

Intermediate MFR Therapist
Innova Physical Therapy, Queensbury, NY
Innovapt.com

*S*hannon Regner, MSPT, is a respected physical therapist who practices in New York. I have known Shannon for four years, have had the pleasure of attending many classes with her, and have seen firsthand her dedication to healing. She specializes in pelvic health related conditions.

J.P: "How did you learn about the JFB-MFR Approach?"

S.R: "I learned about the JFB Approach through another PT who works in Pelvic Health. She recommended the Women's Health course for 'bringing it all together' for practice techniques."

J.P: "What type of therapy were you practicing prior to MFR?"

S.R: "I worked in a hospital based, outpatient orthopedic clinic when I first learned about MFR. I previously used exercise, stretching, massage, and modalities for helping people heal and return to function."

J.P: "Did you learn anything about fascia in grad school?"

S.R: "We did learn about fascia in grad school. Though to become proficient in any particular area of PT, I truly believe one needs to pursue continuing education for additional training. These classes I took outside of grad school helped me improve upon my skills and knowledge base."

J.P: "What impact has MFR had on your life, personally and professionally?"

S.R: "I see MFR help my patients every day in the clinic! Having this tool has opened the door for greater healing and improvements in the population that I treat. I had one patient with bladder pain for many years. We used MFR over her abdomen and an old scar and she felt 100 percent improvement after one session! Another patient with pelvic and back pain due to a fractured pelvis, saw amazing release after MFR treatments. There is something powerful with the MFR approach that patients are able to sense and feel."

J.P: "What is one piece of advice or wisdom you would share with anyone interested in learning more about this approach?"

S.R: "Try it! Feeling the releases and seeing others improve with treatments are the best ways to know if this is a treatment that you want to learn more about."

J.P: "Please share a little bit about your practice and what types of patients you treat. What percentage are Women's Health?"

S.R: "I practice in Queensbury, NY with a focus on pelvic health for women, men, and children. 95% of the clients I treat have some type of pelvic health concern. This may include urinary or bowel incontinence, pelvic/hip/back pain, pelvic organ prolapse, urinary urgency or frequency, prenatal and postpartum issues."

J.P: "How do your patients find you? Are they coming in specifically for Myofascial Release and/or Women's Health?"

S.R: "Most of my patients find me through a Google search when they are trying to find help for their pelvic condition. Other patients are referred by their medical provider or a friend. The majority of patients come in for a pelvic concern and I utilize and educate them on MFR."

It can be difficult when looking for a therapist who offers Myofascial Release in your area. The John F. Barnes Directory of Therapists is a wonderful resource, no matter where you are located. It contains a list of clinics and therapists who have received training in Myofascial Release, under the expert guidance of John F. Barnes himself. You can find this directory at: mfrtherapists.com.

To the Therapists to Come

For all the current Doctors of Physical Therapy students and recent grads, this section is for you! You have an incredible opportunity to learn about the fascial system and incorporate it early on in your careers. I highly encourage you to take a Myofascial Release course immediately after you get your DPT license. It will, hands-down, give you the complete education you didn't get in your graduate program. This is not said to slight your school; it is just the sad fact that science is finally catching up and realizing the significance of the fascial system in relation to the human body. I urge you to realize that some of what you learned in school was incorrect. Be okay with that. Know that we are not linear beings; in fact, there is not one linear thing in the human body. Experience and continued education will be tools in your belt as you continue in your career.

HEALING AT HOME

"Families are the compass that guides us. They are the inspiration to reach great heights, and our comfort when we occasionally falter." –Brad Henry

I could not get educated enough. I began to immerse myself in as many classes as I could. I didn't care about the expense, travel, or if my bosses would reimburse me. I just craved learning more and more, deepening my understanding of the fascial system, this approach and my touch. Soon, I was starting to understand Myofascial Release on a scale that allowed me to practice the techniques at home, both with myself and my family.

Advance Rebounding was a class that became an important piece of my puzzle. Many compressive techniques were presented in this class; one in particular I responded to in a surprising way. This technique was being practiced on me when my leg began to twitch, small, jerking movements at first. I was unaware of why or how I had begun to move. Soon, my leg started to jerk up and down in a rapid, pushing motion. At the same time, my eyes welled with tears. There was no real reason, at that moment, that I could see for my body to react that way. I did not have an emotional thought in my head; I did not have a particularly hard day. I had simply begun to cry while my leg jumped around in front of me. Later, I would realize that I had this reaction because the technique was largely compressive, which stirred up my personal holding patterns, but at the time, these involuntary motions only confused me.

DR. JESSICA L. PAPA

Just as before, the rebounding had stirred up my past trauma and was fighting to force my body to complete its holding pattern. If you watched my session, you would see eerie similarities between what I did on the table and how I fought to free myself from my ex-husband's hold. My legs kicked, my body went tense, my jaw clenched. I went right back to that night, but this time, I walked away free. Really free.

I returned home that night, my experience weighing heavily on me. My key slid into my front door, and instantly, I realized that a switch had been flipped in my head. I was more aware; my senses, once dulled by the monotony of a passionless life, brightened. I could feel the breeze against my skin the way I could not before. Food tasted more delicious, colors were more vibrant. My patience was long suffering when before I had been quick to anger. I couldn't wait to give the same gift to my patients.

I utilized the private treatment room at work for the first time the next day. My patients, once hesitant, became more trusting of MFR, and ultimately, me. In the private room, they were able to give in, mind and soul, to their treatment the way I had. They vocalized their pain and released it into the world; they allowed their traumas to disappear. They, too, found themselves viewing the world, and themselves, in a new light. I was seeing success.

This cemented a decision in my mind. Although I had become much more happy at the clinic I was working in, I wanted so much more. Thoughts of opening my own practice had been floating around in my head for a long time, but logistically I was not quite ready. Instead, I made another change and relocated my services to a new clinic. It was there that I was able to begin practicing MFR almost exclusively.

During all of this, before my Advanced Rebounding class, I attended a course that focused on cervical thoracic techniques and was even more technical than Rebounding. It was the type of class that the left brain craves. Again, I found my left leg twitching chaotically and my body radiating a now familiar heat. My ears pounded, and eventually, tears found their way to my eyes and began to stream down my face. All this was because my partner was holding two pressure points behind my ears, the mastoid processes.

The pressure she applied was gentle, yet it felt like a nightmare. I felt as if she was holding my head and neck down to the table so that I could not move. I later found out that she was not, and I was, in fact, experiencing a fascial response. Everyone is different and will have a different "fascial voice" that is unique to them. Mine feels like I am being suffocated; a pressure pushes against my face and neck as I recall my trauma. Now that I have had treatment, I no longer react the same way, but at that moment, I moved my head side to side, hoping to keep ahead of that pressure.

The lecture portion of the class was just as riveting. I soaked up each word, asked questions and received answers. I wanted to know everything that the instructor knew. I wanted to live and breath MFR. This passion bled into my work. I shared everything I had learned, from the science behind fascial release and the phenomenon that takes place during MFR. My patients listened and received me and MFR well.

Sharing in my professional circles was not enough. My passion soon made its way home. I started to practice therapy on everyone I could get my hands on. First, I purchased a traveling therapy table for home, and allocated time every week to begin treatments on both of my parents. My mom was an instant support, embracing my work from the day I told her about my first class. My dad took some convincing.

At first, he, like many of my new patients, had trouble grasping the concept that mind and body are intrinsically connected. I remember him being so goofy when my mom was getting treated by me; he wanted to talk, and joke, while we were trying to be quiet and centered. His shoulder had been injured at the gym, and that was where I started. His goal was to regain full range of motion and to get back to working out with the same intensity as before, as well as being able to garden again.

I began to give him Myofascial Release Therapy two to three times a week. For six weeks we kept up the routine. He responded very well, surprising himself, just as much as me; 50% pain reduction was achieved during this initial time period. He was hooked. Soon, my Dad was not only managing his pain, but he was finding a reduction in shoulder and neck stiffness that had plagued him even longer than his shoulder injury. Thoracic restrictions were also lessened. As he began to be able to make the connection between his physical well-being and his mental state, he reached more and more goals.

I was surprised after a few sessions how Dad was able to really tune in to what he was feeling. He was a great patient, craved knowledge and instruction. I am very much my father's daughter and I never noticed it as much as I did while treating him.

Growing up, he was a strong male figure in my life. He was the disciplinarian in my family, and I respect him deeply. He taught me about having a work ethic, how to be resilient, and I believe my tenacity comes from him. I distinctly remember one of the most trying days of my early graduate school life. I had come home for Thanksgiving break. I was going through an especially difficult time with my then-partner, and to add to that, final exams were in the near future. I remember after dinner, Dad walked me to my car and packed it up with me. I gave him a final hug goodbye, but had a tough time letting go. I melted down to tears and told him I didn't think I could do it. Through my sobs, I told him I didn't believe that I could actually finish graduate school, that it was too tough.

He said "Little girl, there isn't anything that you set your mind to that you can't accomplish. I know you can do this."

He called me every few days to check in throughout my time at graduate school after that, and was hands down, my biggest cheerleader. I'm so lucky to have a father like him. He has always been there for me, through good times, and not so good times. He is now, as he forever has been, one of my biggest supporters.

Recently, my dad injured his knee painting. Never wanting to bother me, I only caught wind of it from my mom. Of course, I made a house call to treat one of my favorite patients. I get my stubbornness from him, and he tried to convince me that it wasn't so bad and there was no reason to treat him. He might have been right; it was a simple injury, but he was wrong about not treating it. The longer you wait to treat an injury, the longer your fascia has to harden and inflammation to set in. This is when you begin to lose range of motion and long-term damage occurs. After six sessions of therapy, he was as good as new.

Thinking back to my first MFR class, I remember hearing the instructor discuss tissue memory, cellular consciousness, and healing. He talked about how tissue holds memory and that our bodies store that; I couldn't help but think of my mom, on the other hand. I couldn't wait to go home after class and work on her. I was excited to share all that I learned with her now that I felt like I understood her pain so much better.

Until then, no one truly understood the root of her pain. She was always "sick" growing up, and it got tiring for me as a kid to have an excuse for why she couldn't attend school functions, my games, even church. Of course, later I would come to fully understand why she couldn't face going back to church again, but at the time, I was very confused.

I remembered when my brother and I were children she had been very sick. Even into our early adulthood, she was unable to be present in our lives the way a mother should be. She struggled with her diagnosis of Lupus, a systemic disease, as well as fibromyalgia and Rheumatoid arthritis. She was in pain.

She also dealt with a great deal of emotional and physical trauma at an early age. At the time that she had been hurt, situations like hers were stifled, pushed under the rug, in fear of disrupting appearances and familial harmony. She had been robbed of the chance to heal, to find closure. As much as it pains me, I wondered if the abuse she had suffered at the tender age of 15 could be connected to the pain that she struggled with, even then in her middle age.

I was well acquainted with the health concerns of my mother as an adult. Lupus affects your organs and immune system. The resulting symptoms drain you of your energy, strength, and personality. My maternal grandfather had passed when my mother was three years old from his own struggle with Lupus, so she was aware of the genetic possibility she would have it from an early age.

Fibromyalgia can send you into a flare up of intense nerve pain at the slightest touch. These two diagnoses together made for a toxic cocktail in my mother's body. Through my research, I came across a surprising amount of evidence that showed that fibromyalgia is often detected after trauma. My brain began to piece together a picture of my mom: a perfectly healthy teenager being disassembled by that one act of abuse, causing suffering well into her 50s.

The day that her trauma took place, not only was an emotional well-being destroyed, but also her physical health. I saw her crumbling slowly as her body fought to complete the cycle of flight-or-fight, her autonomic nervous system constantly on overdrive. Like dominos, her inability to release the emotional trauma caused the rest of her to fail. Each illness built on the next, until she was incapacitated with pain and discomfort. She was trapped within her own body.

Despite all of this, my mother is one of the kindest, most loving people I have ever met. She struggled through all of this pain and heartache to achieve a Master's Degree in English early on in her life. When she had my brother and I, she stayed home for around six years, earning her Bachelor of Arts in Education at night school. Eventually, she began working in a school district as an English teacher, a position she still has. Through all of this, not many people even knew she was sick. Her passion for teaching overshadowed her bad days, and she was able to bring her all to her work and family in a way that I am still in awe of. She was, and continues to be, an inspiration.

Students flocked to my mother. They saw her as a friend, even more so than an educator. One particular eighth grade student confided in her that she was being abused at home, in a situation that greatly resembled my mother's own traumatic event. My mom immediately jumped into action, ensuring that the student was placed in a safe environment, and was given the help she desperately needed. That day, when my mother came home, memories of her childhood abuse came flooding back. Pushed over the edge, my mom was in a place mentally that she had never allowed herself to be before. She confronted memories and emotions that had been pushed down into a place within her that could not be reached. It was an eruption. She finally asked for help.

After that first class, I finally understood the mind and body connection, and by extension, my mother. I gave her the biggest hug when I got home. The respect I have for her is immense and only grows as I am able to see more and more of what makes her, her. I am so proud of her accomplishments; despite having experienced such a dramatic trauma at a tender age, she is an esteemed teacher, and so much more. Most people would have no clue she was living with so much discomfort. I treated her and she started to unravel; the tears came first, then with craniosacral work, her neck and jaw began to gently release.

The trauma was already so close to the surface that she responded to the therapy immediately. Experiencing her unique response to the therapy, she allowed her voice to be heard. I worked with her utilizing craniosacral work, as well as structured Myofascial Release, always assuring her that I was there for her in every way. She shook and cried, struggled and gained clarity. Her pain lessened and I started to see a change in her, the same way she had seen one in me. Able to allow the cycle of emotional responses to complete, my mother found a new zest for life. Symptoms of her illnesses eased; she had more energy and found her personality returning. I had my mom back. She continues to work on her physical restrictions, as well as the emotional pieces. She realizes that healing is a journey, not a single event, and that her journey is ongoing.

Myofascial Release Therapy was beginning to shape me from the inside out. My body was becoming healthier, and because of it, my mind was becoming stimulated. My family was seeing benefits and my patients were happier. I knew that my path was slowly moving toward extending my passion to my own practice.

BEYOND TECHNIQUE

*F*our years later, I was far away from the hardships of Rhode Island. Beautiful, sunny Sedona, Arizona was as far as you could get in my mind. I was there for my Myofascial Release III, Expert class. To be accepted into this class was truly an honor and a privilege. As a student at the core, I was eager to learn and gain meaningful experiences with other therapists who had found the same passion in Myofascial Release that I had, but the rest of me still held on to a darkness that threatened to diminish all the healing I had found.

MFR III is a class that is mandatory for therapists who wish to advance in the Myofascial Release hierarchy of classes. I had exhausted the resources near me and had decided to take advantage of what was being offered in Arizona. I remember being fairly upset most of the time that I was there. I was not able to totally connect into my power or my feeling intelligent. I was not able to totally let go of the incessant "need to know" what was happening in treatment. Connecting the dots was so important to me for the longest time. I wanted to know why. This was an issue because in MFR, you are taught to truly connect into your right brain during facilitating and receiving treatment.

The right side of your brain is where you express feelings, creativity, and artistic abilities. It is also the place that love, intuition, and thoughtfulness is derived. For me, things were still fragmented. Emotional release for me, at that time, came in the form of tears and deep sadness, with the occasional feeling of anger bubbling under the surface.

I honestly attempted to control my releases for so long, not allowing myself to find release. Finally, one evening in class, I was unable to avoid the inevitable. I surrendered to the therapy, and my mind to the abyss. I gave my body into the right brain way of thinking, feeling and letting go. I so badly needed it. I began to heal once again.

The quivering in my right thigh began. It was a comfort to see my leg jerk up and down; it reminded me of my first Rebounding class and the relief of that session. My nose twitched. My fascial voice started to sound and my head gently turned back and forth. The dreaded tears began to roll. Then, anger. I had expected sadness, bitterness even, as that's what I had received all the other times. But no, red hot anger.

The therapist that was working on me was pushing down on my chest. Inside, I fought. *I hate that!* The voice inside shouted at me. *Stop!* I began to physically recoil, struggling to move away from the technique, to get off the table. Yet, she continued to hold me down. Her hand moved up to my throat and my breathing became more rapid, more frantic. *Why wasn't she stopping?*

The painful heartache from four years before started to crack from within my chest. It felt so real again. I could hear my ex-husband's breath matching mine, his muffled shouting through the pillow. The therapist's hands were no longer hers, they were his. She wasn't trying to heal me, he was trying to suffocate me.

It was as if I was watching a movie. I was the main character, reliving the most horrific night of my life over again. All the terrible thoughts, panicked pleading, and fear resurfaced. It was my body's tissue memory. It was forcing me to live out my incomplete cycle.

The stimulation of compression and energy over my throat, neck, and psoas had catapulted my mind back to that night. During that session, I truly felt trapped, just as much as I did when he had cornered me. The desperation to break free and run was as real as anything I had ever felt.

I thanked God when the session was complete and I was finally released from the hold. I lied there numb and foggy. After, I found my way into the red rocks. I wasn't sure what I was looking for, all I knew was that I needed to clear my head; I needed to be alone. As I walked through the rusty dust, towers of burnt orange rising around me in gentle slopes, I once again found clarity. My senses brightened, my head poked through the clouds. I was achieving balance, yet my heart still felt heavy.

Again, I thought of being in a movie. I could see my character moving closer and closer to the resolution of their story, yet I felt this compulsion to hit pause every few seconds, just before my character could take her next step. I was stuck, frozen in time. I was inadvertently putting the brakes on during my treatments, unable to fully let go, which was holding me back from fully feeling.

Professionally, MFR has given me a tremendous amount of confidence in the workplace. Transforming from feeling unsure about the results my patients had with regards to their treatment to feeling assured that it was my treatment that was making the difference was inspiring. Remarking how confident they felt in my treatment, my patients stated that they could really "let go" in my office. Ready to handle any patient that comes through my door is uplifting.

"You will out-perform all the therapists in your clinic when you go home and return using these new skills," stated John, during many of my classes. He couldn't have been more correct, and boy, did this stir things up for me at work. Here I was, a young Doctor of Physical Therapy in a top-rated outpatient clinic, getting requests from patients, including doctors, to work with me, instead of my boss or other colleagues. Having a two month long wait list and patients coming in from other states left me in high demand.

Noticing that my thinking was continuing to change from strictly linear, logical, detailed and verbal, to a more creative, receptive and balanced thought process was vitalizing. I was learning to let go of old schools of thought that were drilled into my head during graduate school.

I walked away from my MFR III experience with a fully stocked tool belt. Not only was I able to treat patients with better care, I had found some semblance of peace. I was a better therapist and person. I was ready for my next step.

ARANCIA

"If your actions inspire others to dream more, learn more, do more, and become more, you are a leader." -John Quincy Adams

As I became more involved with the practice of John F. Barnes' Myofascial Release Therapy techniques, I realized I was becoming a better therapist. I was reaching patients in a way that I had not thought possible when I was working within the restraints of traditional therapy. After my trip to Sedona, I made a decision. I needed a larger platform, I needed to reach more people in pain. John Barnes says, "You can only take your patients as far as you have been." I believe in this sentiment with my whole being. This did pose an interesting question: now that I had been so far with MFR, who would I be bringing along with me? Arancia Physical Therapy started to form in my mind.

What is in a name? I had made the decision to start my own business and now needed to know what to call it. My first instinct was to call it Matrix Physical Therapy. I wished to start educating my potential clients from the moment they set eyes on my sign, especially on the concept of fascia. I wanted to show how deeply fascia extends and its relationship with the extracellular matrix. So, with a vision board in hand, titled with this name, I met with my next step, an ad agency, Glad Works.

I walked into the bakery we were meeting at with the board and a bag full of fruits. My dad and I had spent hours in Whole Foods the day before, examining all different types of produce. I cut them up in all sorts of ways to demonstrate to the marketing expert what my business would be all about, to show him what fascia was, and how a physical therapy office could use Myofascial Release to heal. At that time, an orange in the hand was just a tool.

Adam, my contact with the agency, and I came up with a plan. We laid out the exact steps I would need to take to make a professional website for this business. I remember nervousness melting away into anticipation with each new step we outlined. This was it, this was the beginning.

I threw myself into the more technical side of the business: finding a physical space to practice, the funding that was needed, and advertising. Something didn't feel quite right. My mind kept returning to the sliced grapefruits and oranges I had hauled into that first meeting. While developing my website, Gina, the owner of Glad Works, sat me down to get a feel for who I am and what I wanted my business to become. I even gave her a treatment, showing her exactly what MFR is and what it can do for people.

It didn't take long for her to voice my own concerns. She explained to me the harsh imagery a name like Matrix PT conjured up, in contrast with the safe, genuine place of healing that I wanted to create. We began to brainstorm. I was explaining to her the concept of fascia and used an orange analogy to describe what fascia is. The fruit flashed through her head once again and she made a suggestion.

"Arancia" is the Italian word for "orange." I let the word roll across my tongue over and over. It hit my ear just right and the fresh, bright feelings it invoked perfectly aligned with the environment I wished to construct in my practice. I knew that I had found a name for the new stage of my life. That afternoon I wrote up the orange analogy that I still use to this day to explain fascia to new clients.

It was 2015, and at that point, I was still finding my way. I was recently divorced and recovering from the struggles I had faced pertaining to that. Living at home with my parents, I was not living an authentic life. Just as discovering MFR had awoken a beautiful passion within me years before, building my business stirred vitality deep down in my being. I began to live my life again. The movie was no longer paused. The hardships I had faced made me appreciate this feeling of renewal that much more.

Even so, I did find a roadblock of my own making: I was fearful. To make Arancia PT a reality, it would mean leaving the security of a full-time job and all the benefits that it afforded me. I was having a difficult time making the leap and was instead trying to work with one foot out the door. I tried to compromise. I started making housecalls, building a business by treating patients at home. I catered mostly to patients that could not leave their homes without great difficulty, including pregnant women who were dealing back and pelvis pain.

I was juggling my job at an established physical therapy office Mondays, Wednesdays, and Fridays, working 13-hour days. On my off time, I was traveling and treating patients. I was also building my client base. It did not take long to become exhausted. Hauling a therapy table in and out of houses gets old after your sixth patient of the day!

I was looking for a place to call home, at least professionally. The first office I took a look at was suggested to me by a current client. It was perfect to start out as a very small operation and I began the process to rent it soon after. It would be prudent to mention that this was by no means easy financially.

At the time, I was living at my parents' home, recuperating from the chaos I had been thrown into over the past few years. My parents initially didn't ask me to contribute, but to my surprise, they eventually did start charging me rent. At first I was more than a little dismayed with the new arrangement, but understood.

I handed over the money with a grimace on my face every single month, wishing it was going into my bank account instead. I was, after all, starting my own business. I admit that I knew that would have probably not have happened anyway; my ability to save was a struggle. But still, it stung.

The day I was to get my keys to the new place, my dad called me into the kitchen just as I had one foot out the door. I didn't want to. I had so much to accomplish before the end of the day, and honestly, I was

DR. JESSICA L. PAPA

extremely busy. The tone of his voice told me that there was no use in arguing so I trudged back in. He and my mom were sitting around the table, looking at me with matching expressions on their faces.

"What's this?" I asked, picking up a white envelope they had placed before me when I sat down.

Dad raised his eyebrow, "Take a look."

My heart was beating so fast when I used my fingernails to tear the top, only to see a sea of green inside. It was every single dollar I had paid them over the past year. They had been saving it for me. My eyes prickled with tears as my tongue searched for the right words.

No business can get started without support. My parents were, and are, exactly that. When I outgrew my initial office and began the search for a new space all over again, they were right back at my side. This time, it was a much longer process.

We looked and looked and looked. There was a former dental office in Warwick, RI that I was particularly fond of, but the structural changes we would need to make were daunting. Then, to my surprise, the current home of Arancia PT came out of an unexpected place. For ten years, my dad had been getting his haircut at a barber in Cranston, RI. While at his visit, he was sad to learn that the barber was retiring that year, but was excited to see a "For Lease" sign in the window on his way out. He called me immediately.

My father had been by my side through every step along my way, thus far. I knew, of course, that I would be able to make this next transition in my professional life no matter what, but it would never have felt right without him; he was my rock through each and every hurdle in my path. After chasing down listings together, checking potential properties for me, and knowing exactly what I needed, he was exactly the person who was meant to stumble across this place.

When I walked in, I knew this was the place we needed to be. There was space to grow, easy construction, it was in a desirable location. I was in love. The purchase went through, not without a few hitches, but within six months, I was the owner and operator of Arancia PT in its current reincarnation. I could not have been happier.

My patients came and I started to take on new ones. We healed together. From my website to my table, Arancia PT has become so much more than an office. It has become a place where passion and healing coexists, bringing relief and understanding to each and every person who enters its doors. When patients come into Arancia, it is my top priority that they feel welcome, important, acknowledged, and cared for. I train my staff to cater to our patients needs. We treat clients as people first, patients second.

When you visit Arancia PT, you will receive individualized, unique care. Pain pills are not our first step; injections and surgery, a last resort. You will take your health into your own hands when you visit me. You will learn how to perform regular self-treatment techniques at home, as explained earlier.

MFR is by no means a quick fix approach. It requires patience and understanding of the body. One must listen to the warnings and red flags the body gives us, and know when and where to treat the symptoms you are feeling. Following the feeling of the symptoms can help lead you to the root cause. Because of this, and as a new patient, you will be seen frequently.

MFR works in succession and builds upon itself. The goal is to reach the deeper structures of connective tissue, all the way down to the cellular level. Again, this is not a quick fix. If treatments begin, and there is a large time lapse in between more treatments, the body will likely go back to the holding patterns it is accustomed to. For this reason, your treatment plan can find you on my table more often than you expect or are used to.

Finding your way to Arancia PT may be a long road, full of bumps and road blocks. We want you to find a home with us where you are treated as a person, more than the sum of your symptoms. We have patients who travel from near and far to receive the care their bodies so desperately need. More importantly, if we can't help you or if we are too far, we will happily find another specialist who can help you. You can also expect that we will follow up with you to be certain that you landed in good hands.

"You Cared, You Shared, You Were Always There"

Gram's Wisdom:

7/6/1917- 3/14/2018

*M*y grandmother was a remarkable woman. She was a combination of warmth and kindness, laughter and love, devotion and wisdom. She encouraged my dreams, overlooked my shortcomings, and praised my every success. I'll never forget how she used to light up when I'd walk in the room. The feeling of being the center of someone's world, no matter how brief, is one of the best on the planet. My Grandma Terry always made me feel that way; I was her happiness and she was mine.

Toward the latter years, it would take her a minute to realize it was me when I visited and when the realization hit, a huge smile would appear on her face, immediately followed by tears of joy. I'd go over, and sit with her, embracing her tightly. Then, I would tell her all about my life. There was no one in the world I was more eager to share with and no one who so fully experienced the highs and lows of my life with me.

Then, when the tears were dry and our days had been discussed, I would begin to treat her with Myofascial Release. She absolutely loved cranial work, and loved to have her arms and legs pulled. I took my time with my favorite patient. When I would finish, it was amazing to see the burst of energy it would give her. Lethargic before my visit, she would perk right up and talk and talk for hours. My Gram seemed years younger, and according to her, felt younger.

Most times after I treated her, she would get very silly. She'd have laughing fits over the littlest things, like breaking wind or if her room-mate said something a little off beat. She just burst into laughter. Her joy truly made me a believer in the saying, "Laughter is the best medicine." After an afternoon and evening of newfound energy, she would tire herself out and get a wonderful, full night's sleep.

Gram looked forward to her treatments and told everyone in the nursing home about her granddaughter. I am proud to say that each and every resident in there knew who I was, and a whole lot of details about me that I probably wouldn't have mentioned myself. I was just as proud of her.

It is fitting that this is the way that we spent our time together at the end of Gram's life. I first became introduced to the field of physical therapy through her. Gram had one pace in life, fast. If she was doing anything, she was doing it quickly and efficiently. She had little patience for slow pokes, and was known for juggling several different projects at once.

Eventually she learned the hard way that fast isn't always the way you want to live your life. Gram was treasurer of the Meadowlarks, a senior citizens club she was a part of, as well as involved with a Rhode Island hospital where she would knit about 100 baby hats for the new-borns every month. She was recognized for her devotion to the hospital Labor and Delivery unit several times. She had many friends and would enjoy going out often. To the age of 88, she was part of a bowling team. Until she fell and broke her hip, her life was busier than mine!

She was a socialite, yet independent, living on her own after her husband passed at the young age of 43. She never remarried. Instead she raised her two daughters on her own, and managed to give them a re-warding childhood, often traveling, and enjoying time with the family.

It was a cold, icy day in March when she fell at a department store parking lot and landed on her right hip. She screamed in pain and I knew immediately that whatever had happened would have dire consequences on her health. I remember the frightened look on her face as she was being wheeled through the doors of the emergency room. She was told by her doctor that she would need to have emergency surgery to include a total hip replacement. My parents and I were there by her side as she underwent the procedure. At the time, we were warned that even though the procedure was in many ways routine, it would be risky for her due to her age.

She survived it and healed well, but would require home care physical therapy and a visiting nurse to come to her home to begin rehabilitation. She was not a big fan of doing exercises, especially because everything was to be done very slowly! She couldn't zip around the house anymore, drive, or bowl. Even sitting in her favorite spot on the couch was off limits due to her range of motion restrictions following surgical post-operative precautions.

My grandmother thought it would be a good idea for me to sit in on her treatment sessions, partly because she was a little nervous and wanted a familiar face at her side, and partly because she thought I may want to see what the physical therapy career was all about. She was right, it piqued my curiosity and at the age of 19, I was rethinking the path my parents so badly wanted me to go down, which was teaching.

At the time, I knew it wasn't for me and I was just going through the motions, but until this point, I didn't have anything better in mind that I wanted to pursue. She must have known me better than I knew myself because I had never really expressed that outloud.

After watching my grandmother go through her rehab for several months, transitioning from home care to an outpatient clinic, I was falling in love with the profession. I decided the next logical step would be to talk to my college advisor, and see about getting me on the track to apply to PT grad school. One minor hitch, I was already in my junior year of college, and very much wanted to graduate the following year.

My Grandmother Terry lived to be 100 years old and left me with much more than memories. Through the years, she spoke about a lot of different things. Love, dedication, healing, and health. I held those words of hers in my heart and soul, a reminder of who she was and who I am because of her. Her wisdom has become a cornerstone of my life, and today, I want to share it with you.

"Regardless of the situation or circumstances it's for the best. Choose a career you love, it will fill your soul. Have money on your own." She said, when I was deciding on college and how my then-boyfriend fit into my plans.

"Everything happens for a reason; it's what you do after it happens that's the true test of your character. Have a good work ethic. Get good at writing things down, track everything. Make a budget." There was a hint of admonishing in her voice when I complained about not having weekends off. She was a bookkeeper and secretary at a well-established law firm in Rhode Island and was always tracking things, keeping a budget and plan, crunching the numbers.

Then, when I cried in her arms when I left my husband, "Don't stay in a bad marriage. Only stay together as long as you're happy."

She taught me how to stay organized, to plan for the future, but most importantly, she was my sounding board. I could tell her anything and she would just listen. She always made me feel like the most important person in her world, and would check in on me regularly. She showed me how to make the roadmap to help me reach my goals. She told me to smile even if it hurts.

There is a quote that I love, "Sometimes you don't feel the weight of what you've been carrying until you feel the weight of its release." I did not fully grasp the meaning of this until I was sitting in my first continuing education course many years after I first began this journey.

It was one of those days in Arizona that are so hot that you feel every ounce of moisture being wicked away by the sun. Excitement and curiosity mingled in my gut as I sat in my chair in the big hotel conference room, listening to the talk on fascial pelvis many, many years after Gram broke her hip. My mind wandered just for a moment and I had that all too familiar gnawing at my upper to mid back. It was like someone was sitting behind me, poking at my muscles with a blade. It was relentless. No matter how I shifted in my seat, it would not go away, it would not let up.

Prior to taking this class, if somebody had told me that with one technique, performed far from where the pain was generating, I would find relief, I would have laughed in their face. At this point, I had tried all sorts of traditional treatment including physical therapy, yoga, massage, and meditation. They all gave me some level of relief, but none that stuck. It wasn't until my first Myofascial Release experience that I found myself walking towards an eventual place of peace, physically and mentally.

Not everyone has come to the same realization, in medicine or outside of it. I have heard it said that "expectations create limitations." It reminds me of traditional therapy, where I first started. Having a preconceived plan of what you're going to do with a patient before you've even seen them on the given treatment day was not the right way to handle patients in pain. I still stand by that.

I have learned that not everyone is coachable or helpable, and that was profound to understand. You can lead a horse to water, but you can't make it drink, as the saying goes- another one of my Gram's. You can't want people to get better more than they want it for themselves. I believe that when a patient walks through my door, they are already halfway there.

What I have discovered through Myofascial Release is what I want for each and every one of my patients. I want the discomforts in their life to no longer weave its way through the fabric of their being, a mystery with no end. I want them to be heard. I want them to see the light in the darkness. I want them to learn the art of healing themselves.

Gram was my finest teacher and my best friend. She led me to where I am in order for me to lead others to a better understanding of not only their bodies, but their emotional well-being, as well. I met pain through watching her suffer and I confronted it when I experienced my own. Now, I conquer it and so can you.

Made in the USA
Las Vegas, NV
07 July 2021